The Cambridge Psychological Library

MANUAL SKILL
ITS ORGANIZATION AND DEVELOPMENT

MANUAL SKILL

ITS ORGANIZATION AND DEVELOPMENT

BY

J. W. COX, D.Sc.

*Research Fellow of the National Institute of Industrial
Psychology, Lecturer in Psychology and Statistical
Methods at the City of London College, sometime
John Stuart Mill Scholar, University College, London*

CAMBRIDGE

AT THE UNIVERSITY PRESS

1934

CAMBRIDGE
UNIVERSITY PRESS

University Printing House, Cambridge CB2 8BS, United Kingdom

Published in the United States of America by Cambridge University Press, New York

Cambridge University Press is part of the University of Cambridge.

It furthers the University's mission by disseminating knowledge in the pursuit of education, learning and research at the highest international levels of excellence.

www.cambridge.org
Information on this title: www.cambridge.org/9781107626126

© Cambridge University Press 1934

First published 1934
First paperback edition 2013

A catalogue record for this publication is available from the British Library

ISBN 978-1-107-62612-6 Paperback

PREFACE

The study of manual skill with which this volume is concerned would seem to require little justification. Facility with the hand has always been an essential factor in human progress. To-day, as in former times, the amenities of life, and even life itself, depend upon man's ability to acquire the manual and other bodily skills necessary to the execution of his ideas. Modern conditions of existence call for a readiness of eye and hand not less than those of the past. If many of our older crafts have now disappeared, this has been offset, in some measure, by the introduction of skills unknown to former generations, and engendered by the same modern machine methods as have done so much to displace the older forms of craftsmanship. The assembling operations which have been selected for special study in this book are a case in point.

In addition to these claims to scientific study on the grounds of its practical importance, manual skill possesses a further and special interest for the psychologist. This it derives from the close connection between manual and mental development. The appearance in man of the higher mental powers which distinguish him from other animals has been largely determined by his ability to develop and to make effective use of the hand. In the early years of the individual, manual control serves as an index to mental growth, the hand constituting one of the chief sources of experience to this end. Various kinds of hand-work have long been recognized in the schools as important educational media.

The present volume, however, will not be concerned with the general problem of mental and manual development, but with problems relating to the acquisition of certain manual skills *after* normal control of the hand has been developed. Nor will it be possible to consider every kind of manual operation, since, for reasons given in the first chapter, an intensive study of a limited region promises more useful results than a more cursory examination of a wider field.

The manual operations here chosen for study are those involved in the manipulation and adjustment of objects to one another. As such, they represent a large and important class. There are, indeed, few skilled operations which do not call for some measure of manipulative skill of this kind. Such operations include not only the use of the hand as a tool, but also the use of tools by the hand, and extend from the simple placing of a lid on a tin, or a nut on a bolt, to the high degree of skill needed by the surgeon.

Even here, however, experimental conditions have necessarily imposed limitations upon the number of operations which it has been possible to investigate. The operations involved in assembling work, together with certain simpler tests of manual dexterity, have been chosen for special study as representing a wide class of manipulative operations.

To study these operations from the point of view of practical measurement will be our first concern. Hence the first step will be to investigate the conditions under which the operations could be employed as tests, and to secure reliable measures of individual ability. The next step will be to investigate the relations between the various measures thus secured. Such measures of ability I have termed 'static functions'; and the investigation of their inter-relations forms the principal topic of the second part of this book.[1] This part will be concerned with the nature of the underlying factors which determine ability at the various operations, and with respect to which individuals may be differentiated and measured. The way in which skill at these manual operations is related to such non-manual activities as mechanical aptitude and general intelligence will also demand careful consideration.

The third step will be to investigate the nature of the changes in ability which are brought about, first by more or less mechanical 'practice', and secondly by a special course of 'training'. Such changes in ability brought about by practice, or by training, I have termed 'dynamic functions'. An examination of their nature, and of their more important relations, will occupy the third part of this book.

The fourth part will be devoted to an account of the mental processes involved in ability and in improvement at the operations. This is based on observations and introspections which were taken throughout the research, and it includes a short excursion into the psychology of shape. The analysis given in this part describes the cognitive activity in manual work. It indicates that mental processes play a larger part in the acquisition of manual skill than is commonly supposed, and provides the basis of the course of training described in the third part.

Briefly, then, I shall consider first the problem of measuring manual skill. Next, I shall consider the nature of the underlying factors which

[1] The first part is introductory in character.

determine its organization. This will be followed by an investigation of the conditions under which manual skill is best developed. Finally, in my analysis, I shall consider an aspect of manual skill which is intimately related to its measurement, its organization and its development.

In concluding this preface, I have many acknowledgments to make. The research was carried out by the aid of a grant made by the Rockefeller Foundation to the National Institute of Industrial Psychology, supplemented by a small grant from the British Association for the Advancement of Science.

The wide programme of testing, practice and training made heavy demands upon the time and attention of my subjects. My best thanks are due to all for so kindly acting in this capacity, and for their detailed observational and introspective notes.

I have also to thank the London and Tottenham Education Committees for permission to carry out work in their schools. To the heads of these schools, Miss M. Manuel and Mr G. H. Thurley, my thanks are specially due for their careful provision of suitable conditions for testing; and also to their staffs for valuable information about the pupils.

Mr V. Gosden, B.Sc., of the staff of the National Institute of Industrial Psychology, has assisted throughout with the calculations and the preparation of the figures for the press. That I can recall only one minor error in all the checking, and sometimes re-checking, to which his figures were subjected, affords the best tribute to the efficiency with which this work has been done.

Anyone who is at all familiar with 'tetrad differences', and with 'fundaments' and 'correlates', will readily appreciate how much certain parts of the research owe to the writings of my former teacher, Professor C. Spearman, F.R.S. But I am alone responsible alike for the conclusions and for the faults of the present research.

Finally, these acknowledgments would be incomplete without an expression of my gratitude to Dr C. S. Myers, F.R.S., Principal of the Institute. The benefit of his wide knowledge and experience has been freely enjoyed by me throughout the research. It was under the stimulus of his encouragement that the training scheme evolved. Every word has been carefully read by Dr Myers before going to press, and the book owes a great deal to his careful editing.

J. W. C.

July 1934

CONTENTS

CHAPTER III

GENERAL PLAN OF THE RESEARCH

Part II. STATIC FUNCTIONS
CHAPTER IV
RELIABILITY

CHAPTER V
THE RELATIONS BETWEEN STATIC FUNCTIONS

CHAPTER VI

THE FACTORS IN 'MECHANICAL' ASSEMBLING

CHAPTER VII

THE FACTORS IN 'ROUTINE' ASSEMBLING

CHAPTER VIII

THE RELATION OF SIMPLE MANUAL TESTS TO THE ROUTINE TESTS

CHAPTER IX

THE MEASUREMENT OF ABILITY AT ASSEMBLING WORK

Part III. DYNAMIC FUNCTIONS

CHAPTER X

ABILITY AND PRACTICE AT 'ROUTINE' OPERATIONS

CHAPTER XI

THE TRANSFER OF 'PRACTICE' EFFECTS

CHAPTER XII

RELATIONS BETWEEN DYNAMIC FUNCTIONS

CHAPTER XIII

THE TRANSFER OF 'TRAINING' EFFECTS

Part IV. ANALYTICAL

CHAPTER XIV

SUBJECTIVE ANALYSIS OF 'MECHANICAL' ASSEMBLING

CHAPTER XV

SUBJECTIVE ANALYSIS OF 'ROUTINE'
ASSEMBLING

Part V. GENERAL SUMMARY

CHAPTER XVI

THE MAJOR CONCLUSIONS AND THEIR SIGNIFICANCE

PART I

THE SCOPE AND PLAN OF THE PRESENT WORK

CHAPTER I

INTRODUCTORY CONSIDERATIONS

A. IMPORTANCE AND VARIETY OF MANUAL OPERATIONS

1. In industry.

Before beginning this investigation, the writer visited a number of factories and studied the work in progress in the various departments. These visits did more than merely convince him of the commonly known fact that a great deal of manual labour is employed in engineering and other forms of factory work. They showed that manual operations, often requiring a high degree of skill, preponderate in many factory departments, and are almost as varied in kind as they are numerous. It was also clear that, although these numerous activities were commonly termed 'manual', they differed considerably in the kind and degree of skill required for their performance. Whereas some could be more or less readily performed by almost anyone, others called for a specially steady hand, a specially light touch, a specially keen eye, or some other special quality of mind or body, and required practice. The operations were also observed to differ with respect to the relative amounts of 'mind' and 'muscle' they seemed to require. In some operations, such as the loading of goods, mere muscle seemed the chief requisite. In others, the necessary manual activity seemed to require fairly complex mental activity which warranted closer psychological study than it had so far received. Of this kind were the assembling operations which enter so largely into the work of the engineering factory, and which form the chief object of investigation in the present volume.

The manual operations of a large factory are divisible into broad classes, according to the general character of the work, as, for example, loading and unloading, sorting, machine-tending, assembling, labelling, packing, etc. It is usual for each class of work to be done in a separate room or department. Thus we have the assembling room, the sorting room, and so on. It is noteworthy that such partition of work is based not primarily on the kind of manual operation it involves, but rather upon the general character of the result.

These broad divisions may usually be subdivided with more regard to the general nature of the work itself. Thus the loading of heavy goods is easily distinguishable, in its demands on the worker, from the loading of light goods, the boxing of chocolates from the boxing of soap tablets, and these again from the packing of the boxes into wooden cases. It is clear that the work of the shop or the factory may include a multiplicity of manual operations and that, although called by the same name, they may involve very different manual activities.

2. IN EDUCATION.

Manual activity can also claim a large and important part in the field of education. In the infant and junior schools, the 'hand' has long been recognized as an important medium for training the mind. In the senior school it continues to play an essential part in the work of the art room, the manual-training centre, the metal workshop, and the domestic science centre. It enters largely into the training of backward and mentally defective children. In many branches of technical education the development of manual skill in relation to some special trade or occupation becomes an important end in itself.

B. PREVIOUS RESEARCH

1. SIMPLE TESTS.

Just as we have seen it erroneous to suppose that manual operations called by the same name, such as 'assembling' or 'packing', necessarily involve the same activities, so it would be equally fallacious to assume, without further inquiry, that an individual's achievement in one manual operation may be taken as a criterion for judging what he would do in another. This could hold only where the abilities concerned have been found to be closely related.[1] Although a good deal of research has already been directed to the investigation of the rela-

---

[1] As shown by the *correlation* between them.

tions between human abilities, previous workers have been more concerned with *mental* than with *manual* operations.

Work on the latter has been limited, in the main, to the simpler manual and sensori-motor tests of the psychological laboratory and to the larger bodily movements. Perrin gave 17 such tests to 51 undergraduates (both sexes) of the University of Texas and found no significant relation between ability at one test and ability at another.[1] Muscio, using tests especially chosen on account of their simplicity, reached a similar conclusion.[2] Some years later Farmer, working with much larger groups of subjects, found a small positive correlation (averaging 0·25) between three sensori-motor tests.[3] He concluded that success at such tests depends upon a common group-factor, associated with the ability to co-ordinate accurately and rapidly the sensory impulses with the muscular movements which they signify. He attributed the difference between his results and those of Perrin and Muscio to differences in the nature of the tests. Shortly afterwards Akroyd, confining his attention to tests of hand and eye co-ordination, found no significant inter-correlation and concluded that each specific combination of movements will require a specific motor test.[4]

Soon after the present investigation was begun, an extensive research into the measurement of manual dexterities was published by Earle and Gaw and their co-workers at the National Institute of Industrial Psychology.[5] They employed tests of relatively simple manual operations not unlike those which had been used previously by Muscio and others, and reached very similar conclusions. The factors which principally determined success in each test were found to be specific to the test situation, so that little could be inferred about a person's ability at other manual operations from his performance at the test. Some of the tests, however, did tend to fall into two groups,

[1] "An experimental study of motor ability", *Journ. Exp. Psychol.* 1921, IV, 24–56. Three of his tests were said to be 'complex', but the complexity consisted in additional *mental* work (e.g. card-sorting, and tracing with both hands simultaneously), not in greater complexity of movement such as is introduced into the tests used in the present work.

[2] "Motor capacity with special reference to vocational guidance", *Brit. Journ. Psychol.* 1922, XIII, 157–84. His tests included aiming, tapping, tracing, simple form board, inserting matches into holes, steadiness and 'total strength'.

[3] "A Group-factor in sensori-motor tests", *Brit. Journ. Psychol.* 1927, XVII, 327–34. The sensori-motor tests were the choice reaction test, the McDougall-Schuster dotting test, and the pursuit-meter test.

[4] "Some tests and correlations of hand and eye co-ordination", *The Forum of Education*, 1928, VI, No. 2, 127–43.

[5] *The Measurement of Manual Dexterities*, N.I.I.P. Report No. 4, 1930.

according to whether 'speed' or 'accuracy' was the main requirement, although the differences were not statistically significant.

2. LIMB AND BODY MOVEMENTS.

Outside the region of simple manual and motor tests, previous research in the field of motor abilities has been chiefly concerned with the larger bodily movements. Such were some of the tests used by Muscio,[1] and many employed by Garfiel.[2] The usual aim of these investigations has been to determine whether there exists a general motor ability common to all motor performances in virtue of which a person who excels in one will tend to excel in all others. If this be so, it would obviously simplify the problems of selection and of organization of workers.

Investigators are not in general agreement on this point. Some, like Perrin and Muscio, deny the fact of a general motor capacity, while others claim to have proved its existence. Garfiel concludes that we *may* rightly speak of a general motor ability[3]: but the many negligible correlations between her tests, and the lack of any suitable criterion for determining the statistical significance of her data, fail to justify this view. It appears to be based largely upon the inadequate fact of low correlation between motor tests and intelligence tests.

The absence of correlation between many motor performances renders it improbable that *all* such performances will depend upon the same common ability (or, more correctly, 'factor'). Nevertheless, the application of the necessary statistical criterion has sometimes indicated a factor running through a restricted group, as in the 'reaction-time' experiments of Rao and of Reymert.[4] The small correlations found between manual dexterity tests by Earle were similarly explicable by a single common factor,[5] though whether this was specifically 'motor', or whether it was the wider factor found in mental performances generally,[6] was indeterminable from the available data.

[1] *Op. cit.* p. 3.
[2] "The measurement of motor ability", *Arch. Psychol.* 1923, No. 62. Miss Garfiel's tests included hand-tapping, foot-tapping, aiming at a target, and various arm and leg movements.
[3] *Op. cit.*
[4] See C. Spearman, *The Abilities of Man* (London: Macmillan, 1927).
[5] *Op. cit.* p. 3.
[6] The '*g*' of Spearman's theory.

C. SOME ASPECTS OF FURTHER RESEARCH

1. THE MEASUREMENT OF ABILITY.

Our examination of previous work indicates several broad lines along which further inquiry may profitably follow. The first of these relates to measurement. Our conclusions about the way in which abilities are related to one another will depend upon observed relations between measurements of the abilities made on individuals. In the field of motor activity such measurements will be usually provided by motor tests, and the conclusions will depend, ultimately, upon the scores made at the tests. Owing to the complexity of mental life, such scores will seldom provide a pure measure of the operation which the test has been designed to measure[1]. On the contrary, various influences affecting the score will tend to intrude which are not an essential constituent of the ability one sets out to measure. While such influences may themselves provide interesting objects of study, it is important to distinguish them from the ability one wishes to measure, and to keep a careful check on the errors of measurement to which they may lead.

These influences have been discussed at length elsewhere.[2] Some occur accidentally and so tend to be distributed randomly through the test. As they may be either positive or negative in their effects, they tend to diminish, by mutual cancellation, as the measure becomes more exhaustive. Other influences follow a more or less regular course. The chief of these arise from fatigue and from practice. Although they can hardly be eliminated, they can be kept under careful observation and control.

The extent to which a test score may be relied on to provide a satisfactory measure is indicated by the correlation between one part of the total score and another, or between the total score and another similarly obtained. Where this 'reliability coefficient' is high, the measure is at least consistent with itself. Before concluding that abilities are unrelated, it is important to ensure that the lack of correlation is not due to unreliable measures. For this reason we have devoted a good deal of attention in the present research to the reli-

[1] 'Pure' in the sense of yielding a constant measure of some static 'ability'.
[2] J. W. Cox, *Mechanical Aptitude: its existence, nature and measurement,* Chapter VI (London: Methuen and Co. 1928).

ability of measurement, and to the conditions affecting reliability. Apart from its bearing on the practical value of the tests, this precaution seemed especially desirable in a field where inter-correlations in the past have been found to be low.[1]

In manual as in most other motor operations, practice usually brings about a large improvement. The effects of practice on the *measures* of these operations will, therefore, merit consideration.

2. THE DEVELOPMENT OF MANUAL SKILL.

The effect of practice on *ability* also calls for further attention. For practical purposes one wishes to know the proficiency to which the testee may eventually attain, rather than his ability at first. Little evidence has been obtained hitherto, in respect of manual operations, to show how far initial ability will serve as a reliable index of ultimate proficiency. To provide information on this, and on such other aspects of ability as may be indicated by the rate of progress made under standard conditions of practice, and by variability of performance, has been a further aim of the present book.

Another aspect of the present inquiry relates to the manner and conditions under which skill in manual operations may be developed. Previous research in this direction has been concerned almost wholly with simple motor activities, such as speed of tapping,[2] or with occupations, like typing[3] and telegraphy,[4] in which the movements are again simple and the learning is largely dependent on non-motor elements.[5] The present inquiry has extended into more complex movements and has carefully distinguished between two broad conditions under which manual skill may develop. In one case, the worker repeats the operation, more or less mechanically, at maximum speed; in the other case, he receives instruction from some competent person. Following the

---

[1] A precaution not always taken in previous work. Perrin gives no reliability coefficients, Muscio only three, Garfiel only in some cases, and these are often low. On the contrary, Akroyd and Earle (*op. cit.*) carefully determined the reliability of their tests, and Akroyd investigated the influence of practice on the inter-correlations.

[2] A. I. Gates and G. A. Taylor, "An experimental study of the nature of improvement resulting from practice in a motor function", *Journ. Educ. Psychol.* XVII, No. 4, pp. 226–36.

[3] W. F. Book, *The Psychology of Skill, with Special Reference to its Acquisition in Typewriting* (New York and London: Gregg Publishing Co. 1925).

[4] W. L. Bryan and N. Harter, "Studies in the physiology and psychology of the telegraphic language", *Psychol. Review*, 1897, IV, 27–33.

[5] E.g. learning the positions of the keys, the Morse code, etc.

usage of C. S. Myers[1], we have called the former method 'practice' and the latter 'training'. So far as the writer is aware, the development of a formal course of training and the investigation of its effects under controlled conditions have not been previously attempted in the sphere of motor activity. That the two methods of acquiring skill differ in important ways is clearly indicated in the results to be described later.

3. THE TRANSFER OF MANUAL SKILL.

Closely bearing on the problem of the development of manual skill is that concerning its transference: how far does the skill acquired in one operation transfer to other operations? Here, again, attention in the past has been focused on simple activities, and the conditions investigated, so far as they relate to motor activity, have been those of 'practice'.[2] The results have shown that, under those conditions of learning, little, if any, transference occurs.

Important differences in the transference effects of different methods of training have been observed in such non-manual and purely cognitive operations as the memorizing of poetry and of nonsense syllables,[3] and the acquirement of ideals.[4] The problem appears never to have been pursued in the region of motor activity. In the well-known dart-throwing experiment of Judd, the training consisted in instruction in the principles of the refraction of light, not in methods of throwing as such.[5] The influence of training methods on the transfer of skill seems especially worth investigating in the more complex and highly skilled movements with which we shall be concerned, both on account of its bearing on educational doctrines in an unexplored field, and in view of the practical problems associated with the transfer of workers from one operation to another, which frequently arise in industry.

[1] "Educability", *Journ. Scientific Transactions*, Brit. Ass. for Adv. of Science, 1928.

[2] Cf. the tapping test and procedure of Gates and Taylor (*op. cit.*), the chain-assembling operation and procedure of J. N. Langdon and E. M. Yates, "An experimental investigation into transfer of training in skilled performances", *Brit. Journ. Psychol.* 1928, XVIII, pp. 422–37, and the card-sorting tests of W. H. Pyle, "Transference and interference in card-distributing", *Journ. Educ. Psychol.* 1919, X, 107–10.

[3] H. Woodrow, "The effect of type of training upon transference", *Journ. Educ. Psychol.* 1927, XVIII, 159–72.

[4] By Ruediger and Squire, see E. L. Thorndike, *Educational Psychology*, II, 411–12.

[5] Subjects were practised at throwing darts at a target below water. When the depth of the water was altered, those who had received instruction in the principles of light refraction quickly surpassed the others. See E. L. Thorndike, *op. cit.* pp. 400–1.

4. THE ORGANIZATION OF MANUAL SKILL.

Another aspect of the present inquiry is concerned with the way in which skill at one manual operation is related to skill at other manual operations. The solution of many practical problems depends on such knowledge. The successful use of vocational tests, for example, rests on a knowledge of the relation between the skill required in the test and that involved in the occupation in which the testee will subsequently engage. Similarly, any attempt to organize manual work along psychological lines must pay due regard to the relations existing between the various operations it is proposed to divide among the workers.[1]

In the present volume we shall extend our inquiry from the simpler tests, which have already engaged the attention of previous workers, to the more complex manual operations of the assembling room, and shall attempt to discover how these operations are related to one another, and to the simpler tests.

In addition to this difference in complexity, assembling operations exhibit other important features which make it impossible to apply to them the conclusions of previous research. Many involve the use of both hands and the performance of several activities simultaneously. All involve the fitting together of objects in such a way that accuracy of movement, as well as speed, is essential to success. In the rigidity of the material with which they deal, and in their well-defined externally-controlled aim, they differ from other kinds of work, such as drawing, painting and the plastic arts generally.

In certain circumstances assembling work may involve more than the manual activity required to assemble the parts; it may present a problem in the relative order and positions occupied by the parts when assembled. Work which thus includes a *mechanical problem* we have termed 'mechanical' assembling. Where no such problem is involved we have called it 'routine' assembling.[2] To inquire into the relation between these two kinds of work is another aim of the present investigation.

Where the correlation between two performances is positive we may assume some common cause, or influence, to account for the correlation; but, unless the correlation is perfect, it would be clearly wrong to suppose that the performances function exactly alike. The measure-

---

[1] More precisely, their *functional* relations.
[2] A term suggested by C. S. Myers.

ment of one, in an individual, will not provide a measure of the other. The ultimate aim in investigating the relationships between the performances should be to discover the nature of the unitary underlying causes which bring about the observed relationships, for these are the ultimate elements in terms of which mental operations may be analysed and measured. For this reason it has seemed desirable to pursue this part of our inquiry beyond the 'abilities' into the 'factors' which determine success in regard to them.

Provided psychological processes are not mistaken for chemical reactions, this aspect of our work may be compared with the analysis of the chemist. Starting with the mineral substances, as presented by nature, his early efforts were to classify them according to such general properties as he was able to observe. Before the development of the experimental method, his observations were largely confined to their more obvious physical properties, such as colour and hardness, with the result that he was apt to place too much reliance on mere *appearance*. Consequently, substances chemically identical, such as water and steam, were regarded as essentially different, while other substances, such as ice and quartz, though composed of entirely different materials, were, owing to their similarity of appearance, looked upon as forms of the same substance. This stage of chemistry is comparable with the sort of psychology open to the non-experimental observations of crude 'common-sense', which is apt to suppose that all activities which have been given the same general name—as, for instance, 'dexterity'—are psychologically identical.

Solid progress in chemistry was only achieved after the development of the experimental method. As a result of carefully planned experiments, knowledge of the true chemical properties of substances was gradually acquired. By this means the elements were eventually distinguished from one another. Such experimental analysis corresponds to the attempt to isolate 'factors' as proposed above.

Having experimentally isolated the 'factors', there remains the complementary task of determining how they function when operating together. Previous researches have already disclosed two factors, namely 'general intelligence' ('g') and 'mechanical aptitude' ('m'), whose presence in certain of the assembling operations seems not unlikely. Consequently, the way in which these function, together with such 'motor' factors as may be discovered, will merit careful inquiry.

Failure to distinguish the abilities, as measured by tests, from the underlying common factors would sometimes account for the divergence of opinion respecting the nature of motor ability observable in previous research, especially where the relation of 'motor' tests to 'general intelligence' is in question.[1] A further source of divergence may be found in the absence of any satisfactory basis for the subjective analysis and classification of motor tests. Such analysis, in terms of unitary mental processes, forms an important parallel inquiry to the objective analysis of 'abilities' in terms of factors. We shall, therefore, conclude the present chapter by some introductory considerations respecting this subjective aspect of the present work.

5. THE SUBJECTIVE ANALYSIS OF MANUAL OPERATIONS.

(a) *Failure to differentiate between operations.* Although much useful introspective work has been carried out in the region of manual activities, a universal weakness where analyses have been attempted would appear to lie in the fact that they seldom penetrate beyond the descriptive level. A typical example is the common classification of motor tests into 'speed' tests and 'accuracy' tests. While these broad differences may for some purposes be usefully distinguished, they afford no logical basis of classification, for these two classes are not mutually exclusive. On the contrary, they are entirely overlapping, for all 'speed' tests need some degree of accuracy, and all the so-called 'accuracy' tests must be carried out with some reference to time. Introspection shows that even in such a typical 'speed' test as 'tapping' much of the effort is expended in regulating the force, direction and positions of the taps—'accuracy' qualities which are ignored in any device for merely recording the number of taps, but which are readily observed when a pianist, for example, strikes the wrong note, or when a very young child is asked to do the 'tapping' test, or when the shapes of dots made at maximum speed with a pencil on paper by different individuals, especially by children of different ages, are compared.

The attempt is sometimes made to distinguish certain motor operations by the fact that they require 'muscular control'. But with this we are no better off than with 'accuracy', for all motor operations involve

---

[1] Thus Abelson, Burt, Bagley, Gesell, Bolton, Kirkpatrick, Wooley, and Fischer find a positive relationship; Clark, Wissler, Binet and Vaschide, Glenn, Perrin, and Gilbert discover no relationship; Terman, Bickersteth, and English assert a negative relation.

'muscular control'. Even in such a mechanical operation as walking, one has only to close the eyes to realize the important part played by control, and the briefest observation of the infant trying to achieve this feat is sufficient to indicate the complexity of the factors that must be 'controlled' before success is achieved. Indeed, if, as seems reasonable, we regard those movements as most highly controlled which have been learnt so well that they have become automatic, the very operations which are said specially to involve muscular control would often be just those in which such control is least developed. What appears to differentiate many operations is not the mere presence or absence of muscular control but the extent to which such control has become automatic. But, even as thus stated, it still provides no psychological basis for distinguishing one kind of motor operation from another, for all tend to pass into the automatic stage with practice.

This common feature of all training goes far to nullify, as distinct groups, the three classes of skilled movement postulated by F. N. Freeman,[1] namely, (a) that in which the connection has to be made between important features of the external situation and movements which are already under control, (b) that which demands the organization of new movements in response to the appropriate features of the external situation, and (c) that in which the series of movements is more complex and the stimulus to which the response is made is more highly organized. With practice the new movements would tend to come under control and so cease to be classifiable under (b) or (c). Such a classification is one of persons[2] rather than of movements. The two additional variables, viz. complexity of movement and organization of stimuli, introduced into (c), provide yet further difficulties, since some variations in complexity of both movements and stimuli must occur in all three classes. If Freeman's three classes of movements be retained and we divide the stimuli into merely two classes, 'simple' and 'complex', we get, at once, by associating each kind of stimulus with each class of movement, six classes of skill.

S. Wyatt[3] analyses the activities involved in soap-wrapping into: (a) finger dexterity, (b) accuracy of movement, (c) rapidity of movement, (d) sensitivity to touch. It is difficult to discover any psycho-

---

[1] *How Children Learn* (London: Harrap, 1919).
[2] I.e. as regards their stage of practice.
[3] "An experimental study of a repetitive process", *Brit. Journ. Psychol.* xvii, 192–208.

logical principle underlying this classification, for 'accuracy' and 'rapidity' together constitute 'dexterity', and what has been said above about 'speed' and 'accuracy' is likewise applicable to 'dexterity'. 'Sensitivity to touch' is, of course, psychologically distinguishable from 'dexterity'—so much so, that its classification as a co-ordinate 'activity' seems very questionable. Such sensitivity provides one of the *classes of experience* in the light of which movements are carried out, and, as such, relates to the cognitive aspect of the activity rather than to the activity itself.

Another type of classification frequently employed is that adopted by Miss E. Garfiel.[1] Her tests are classified into those of (*a*) speed, (*b*) co-ordination, (*c*) steadiness, (*d*) strength and (*e*) adaptability. Of these qualities, 'speed' we have already examined. 'Co-ordination', being merely another aspect of 'muscular control',[2] appears equally ineffectual as a basis for classification for reasons already given in our discussion of 'muscular control'. 'Steadiness', in like manner, results from 'co-ordination' and 'control'; and is, consequently, unable to supply another co-ordinate basis of classification. 'Strength'[3] refers to the force with which a movement is carried out. Seeing that all movements imply some degree of force, they all require some degree of strength. Moreover, the same movement may be carried out with different degrees of force and so require varying degrees of strength.[4] As a *quantitative* attribute of all movements it offers no means of distinguishing *qualitatively* between them.[5] 'Adaptability' refers to the facility for learning the movements rather than to the sort of movements learnt. Since all movements must at first be 'learnt' (in the widest sense of the word), all require, in some measure, adaptability, so that here, again, we are provided with no clearly distinguishable feature whereby movements may be differentiated as to kind.[6]

[1] *Op. cit.* p. 4.

[2] For example, the 'control' of (say) two muscles is a necessary condition of their being 'co-ordinated'.

[3] Subsequently omitted by Miss Garfiel as a 'factor' in 'motor ability'. *Op. cit.*

[4] Compare, for example, the unscrewing of a loose nut with the unscrewing of a tight nut.

[5] A test is commonly said to require 'strength' when it calls for a *high degree* of force. Such usage is, of course, still *quantitative* and *relative*: what might require strength (in this sense) in a child might not in a man.

[6] I.e. as to the psychological processes involved. Usually a test is said to require 'adaptability' when the 'intellectual' aspect of the test seems distinguishable from its 'motor' aspect, as in Miss Garfiel's 'tricks'. Apart from the possibility that such a distinction, on closer analysis, may prove untenable, this sort of 'adaptability' obviously refers to the learning and not to the movements learnt.

(*b*) *Failure to distinguish the activity from its effect.* Another weakness in certain of the foregoing analyses is their failure to distinguish between the movements involved in the operation and the ultimate effect of those movements on the thing operated upon. Thus, when a test is given in such a form that it can only be scored quantitatively, as in tapping or in threading beads, it is classified as a 'speed' test; where qualitative differences are recorded in the work done, as in cutting out a circular disc, the test becomes one of 'accuracy'.

(*c*) *Failure to explain.* A further weakness in current analyses is their failure to offer any psychological explanation as to how various motor operations are effected. To say, for example, that walking involves 'muscular co-ordination' amounts to little more than saying that it involves using the right muscles at the right time. What the processes are which enable us to do this we are never told.

When it comes to explaining how improvement is brought about, the concepts which we have examined are usually replaced by others. Thus, improvement has been said to depend on 'bodily set' or 'upon the ability to maintain a kind of kinaesthetic orientation'.[1] Seeing that we are nowhere told what the processes involved in such an 'orientation' or 'set' are, such statements hardly do more than explain the obscure by the more obscure: and even if this knowledge were vouchsafed us, there would still remain to be explained how such orientation is acquired. The same remark applies to the explanation which imputes progress to 'the acquisition of working methods and techniques'.[2] The important point is to know how these are acquired.

More often than not, we are spared even the above meagre attempts at some positive explanation, and learning is regarded as being largely at the mercy of chance; hence the method of 'trial and error', or, as it is sometimes called, 'trial and success'.[3] In this connection, Professor Pear has already said that "it should not hastily be concluded that such trials must be, because they *are, blind*".[4] On closer analysis, one may perhaps go even farther and say that, in so far as true learning occurs at all, it is never entirely blind.

[1] F. L. Goodenough and C. R. Brian, "Certain factors underlying the acquisition of motor skill in pre-school children", *Journ. Exp. Psychol.* 1929, XII, 127–55.
[2] Cf. A. I. Gates and G. A. Taylor, "An experimental study of the nature of improvement resulting from practice in a motor function", *Journ. Educ. Psychol.* 1926, XVII, 235.
[3] By F. N. Freeman, *op. cit.* pp. 133 ff.
[4] In *Skill in Work and Play*, pp. 37–42 (London: Methuen, 1924).

(*d*) *Failure to indicate psychological processes.* But, perhaps, the most serious weakness in current analyses is that the activities into which motor operations are resolved, or upon which they are said to depend, are not processes at all. Thus 'speed', 'accuracy' and 'steadiness' are obviously not processes underlying movement, but qualities of a movement dependent upon its spatial and temporal characters. Similarly, 'co-ordination' and 'control' are psychological characters which a movement may possess in virtue of its relation to other psycho-physical processes; they offer no indication of the processes whereby such characters are acquired.

(*e*) *The kind of analysis needed.* Enough has been said to indicate the urgent need for a more penetrating and systematic analysis of the operations involved in motor activity than has yet been attempted. Such an analysis should distinguish the objective characters of a movement from the movement itself, and should not confuse the activity which sustains the movement with the physical results achieved by the movement (the work done), nor with the stimulus in response to which the movement is made. It should also distinguish between that part of the activity which is physiological and that which is psychological. Above all, it should aim at resolving the latter into ultimate, unitary, mental processes.

Not only would this type of analysis greatly add to our theoretical knowledge, but it would also prove of great practical service in offering a more scientific basis for the classification of existing motor tests. It would indicate the lines along which new motor tests should be constructed and the direction along which further research on motor activity would most fruitfully proceed. Moreover, it would supply a scheme of reference according to which all the various motor operations underlying skill in work and in games could be analysed, comparable to the tables used by the analytical chemist. Such a scheme would supply the qualitative supplement to the quantitative analysis of the kind suggested on p. 9.

CHAPTER II

GENERAL SCOPE AND METHODS

A. THE OPERATIONS INVESTIGATED

1. GENERAL CHARACTER OF THE OPERATIONS.

We saw, in the last chapter, that the more complex manual operations had hardly received the attention of previous investigators which their importance alike in industry and in education would seem to merit, and that an extension of our knowledge in this direction might lead to results of great theoretical and practical value. Accordingly, it was decided to concentrate the present inquiry on these more complex activities and, for reasons given below (p. 16), to select for special study in this region those operations that are associated with engineering assembling work.

It was, of course, impossible to examine the whole range of assembling operations in the intensive way we desired. It became necessary to choose a limited group which, by including a diversity of movements involving varying degrees of complexity and of skill, would be broadly representative of the many other manual operations observable in assembling and other occupational activities. It was further desirable that the activities chosen should lend themselves to employment as measures of ability under test conditions.

Choice fell upon the various operations involved in the assembling of an electric lampholder as best fulfilling these requirements. Consequently the assembling tests employed in the present research have been built up around the electric lampholder, each involving one of the steps necessary to its assembly. Further diversity and differentiation as regards complexity were introduced by using the same material, first as an 'assembling' test, in which the various pieces have to be put together, and next as a 'stripping' test, in which the assembled pieces have to be taken apart. It will be seen, from the description given in the following chapter, that they include operations which differ widely in difficulty, from the simple screwing in of a screw to the complete wiring up of the holder. For descriptive purposes we shall refer to these as the 'complex' operations in the present study.

We have already had occasion to notice, in Chapter I, that assembly work may sometimes include the solution of a mechanical problem, and we have called such work 'mechanical' assembling in order to distinguish it from 'routine' assembling in which this problematic part is absent. Since both kinds of assembling work are to be found in industry, and the relation of 'mechanical' assembling to such purely mental abilities as 'mechanical aptitude' and 'general intelligence', on the one hand, and to manual abilities, on the other, raises many important questions, it was decided to include both 'mechanical' and 'routine' assembling operations within the group selected for special study. The mechanical assembling tests were also built up around the electric lampholder,[1] in the way described in our next chapter, and they employed the same material as the routine tests. Briefly, then, the assembling operations here studied divide into (i) mechanical assembling operations, and (ii) routine assembling operations; and the latter again subdivide into (*a*) assembling operations, and (*b*) stripping operations. These will form our central object of study in relation to the problems raised in Section C of our last chapter.

For analytical purposes we shall compare the assembling operations with three further broad groups of tests, as explained in Section B below. Two of these groups, namely (*a*) tests and other measures of general intelligence, and (*b*) tests of mechanical aptitude, will measure important aspects of *mental* ability, while the third, which we shall refer to as (*c*) simple manual tests, will be concerned with *manual* operations. For the first group we shall use such customary measures of intelligence as 'reasoning', 'opposites', 'analogies', 'sentence completion' and similar tests, together with suitable measures of ability at school subjects when available; for the second group we shall employ tests which have been developed and described by the present writer in a previous research on 'mechanical aptitude';[2] for the third group we shall take some of the tests of simple operations which have entered largely into previous research, such as threading beads, placing rings over rods and turning screws.[3]

2. REASONS FOR CHOOSING ASSEMBLING OPERATIONS.

The reasons which led us to direct our attention to the more complex manual activities have already been stated. The following considerations determined our choice of assembling operations:

---

[1] Apart from a few additional tests which were sometimes employed.
[2] *Op. cit.* p. 5.   [3] Descriptions of these tests will be found in Chapter III.

(i) The importance of keeping a close check on accuracy of measurement, especially where, as in manual tests, large practice effects might be expected, was referred to in Chapter I. Our measures of the various functions to be observed will themselves need careful examination before we can employ them with any degree of assurance. It seemed, therefore, desirable to preface our inquiry by a more intensive study of the problem of measurement than could have been made over a wider field.

(ii) The restriction of our inquiry to assembling operations also allowed more attention to be given to its subjective aspect. A careful analysis of one field of activity might well indicate the general principles to be followed in other fields. On account of the wide range of activities they embrace, assembling operations provide a good starting point for this purpose.

(iii) The important part which assembling work occupies in industry provided another reason for concentrating on assembling operations. There is urgent need of tests which will gauge a person's suitability for this work, and, consequently, an urgent need of a clearer understanding of the factors which determine such suitability.

(iv) Finally, although differing in many respects, assembling operations also possess many points of resemblance. They all depend upon skilful and rapid movements of the fingers, in which sight and touch play a guiding part. They all consist in bringing external objects into correct spatial adjustment with one another. The general character of the material with which they deal is similar throughout. In these respects assembling operations seemed to fall into a class of their own, whose study might lead to fruitful results for vocational guidance and selection.

B. THE FUNCTIONS TO BE MEASURED

1.. 'FUNCTION' AS DISTINGUISHED FROM 'FACTOR'.

Before discussing the 'functions' which we shall need to measure, it will make for clearness to distinguish the meaning of this term from that of 'factor', with which it is apt to be confused and which we shall also have occasion to use. By 'function' we shall mean any immediately observable performance as it occurs in its concrete entirety. As such it will usually be directly measurable. An example is a person's performance at an 'intelligence' test, as measured by the whole of his score at the test. This performance (and score) will be the resultant of various determinants, such as the influences to which we have already referred,[1] and the facility with which the individual is able to carry out the mental operations involved in the test. Such determinants may, in the popular sense of the word, be called 'factors'. For scientific purposes, however, it is clearer to denote these in general by the term 'influences', and to reserve the term 'factor' for such of them as may be found to operate in systematic and unitary fashion. In this sense the subject's innate ability for mental work in general, and his innate ability for the particular operation involved in the test, would be *'factors'*; his attitude to the test, state of mental fatigue, and similar determinants would remain *'influences'*;[2] and his actual performance would be a *'function'* of all these. Such usage conforms appropriately[3] with that of mathematics; since when we refer to one quantity as a 'factor' of another, we are thinking of its relation, *as a unitary whole*, to this other quantity.

2. 'STATIC' AND 'DYNAMIC' FUNCTIONS.

We may further distinguish between those functions which are conceived as absolute entities, such as a person's initial ability at a given operation or his ability after any given length of practice, and those which relate to changes in these, such as the amount of improvement brought about by practice. The former sort we shall call 'static', and the latter 'dynamic'. The dynamic functions are themselves divisible into those which relate solely to *quantity of change*, irrespective of the time taken to effect it, and those which are further determined by the time taken in effecting the change, i.e. which relate to *rate of change*. Such functions may themselves determine more complex functions; e.g. 'improvability' will clearly depend on the static function 'initial ability', and on the dynamic functions 'total amount of improvement possible' and 'rate at which improvement can be effected'.

3. FUNCTIONS TO BE MEASURED IN ANALYSING 'MECHANICAL' ASSEMBLING.

Where, as in what we have called (p. 16) 'mechanical' assembling, the parts have not only to be put together but their relative positions

---

[1] *Supra*, p. 5.

[2] In a good test such 'influences' would, of course, be reduced to a minimum.

[3] 'Appropriately', because the elucidation of factors can only be effected by mathematical measurements.

have also to be thought out as part of the same complex operation, the latter may be divided into (*a*) a 'problematic' part concerned with the 'thinking out', and (*b*) a 'motor' part concerned with the 'putting together'. The latter seems best measured by the individual's performance at the same assembling work after it has been stripped of its 'problematic' part by ensuring that the individual thoroughly understands how the parts are to be fitted together. The 'problematic' part obviously cannot be measured as an assembling operation independently of the 'motor' part, but by comparing the individual's performance initially with his performance at the same assembling operation after the manner of assembling has become clear, the extent to which the two parts have respectively entered into the initial performance may be estimated. With this purpose in view we have employed the same tests first as measures of 'mechanical' assembling and subsequently as measures of 'routine' assembling.

Previous research goes to show that all intellectual operations are partly dependent on one and the same 'general common factor', which may be isolated and measured; and that where an understanding of mechanical arrangements is needed there is also a 'mechanical', factor. The question, therefore, arises as to how far the mechanical (i.e. the 'problematic') part of assembling work is dependent on these two factors. If it were found to be resolvable into them[1], we should confirm and strengthen our theoretical knowledge of the relations between mental 'abilities' and, at the same time, secure a more direct means of measuring these mechanical assembling operations. To answer this question we must compare ability at 'mechanical' assembling tests with that at 'general intelligence' and 'mechanical aptitude' tests.

To sum up, in order to determine for both theoretical and practical purposes the measurable factors upon which success at 'mechanical' assembling depends, we must compare ability at the following kinds of tests, viz. 'general intelligence' tests, 'mechanical aptitude' tests, 'mechanical' assembling tests and 'routine' assembling tests.

4. Functions to be measured in analysing 'routine' assembling.

In 'routine' assembling the worker is restricted to the manual side of the operation. Seeing that the weight of previous evidence favours

---

[1] Theoretical considerations suggest the likelihood of 'specific' factors also.

the belief that manual work depends upon a large number of unrelated activities rather than upon a *unitary* 'motor' factor, the interesting question here is how far this is true of the more complex operations involved in 'routine' assembling. Is there a 'general routine assembling' ability or, on the contrary, a number of independent 'routine assembling' abilities? The answer has an obvious and immediate bearing on practice, since the mode of procedure to be adopted in estimating an individual's suitability for this kind of work must vary according to which view we accept. To answer it, we must compare abilities at various 'routine' operations.

Such comparison will, however, provide no information as to what are the unitary, measurable, factors upon which success at these operations depends and into which they may be analysed. Although the underlying activity has been referred to above as 'manual', subjective analysis shows that a large number of cognitive operations are involved—though of a different kind from those in 'mechanical' assembling. Hence, theoretical considerations make it important to inquire whether the above-mentioned 'general factor', which seems to run throughout the cognitive operations involved in general intelligence tests, also extends its influence to the cognitive operations in 'routine' assembling.[1] This necessitates a comparison with ability at 'general intelligence' tests.

Again, analysis shows that the cognitive operations of 'routine' assembling are chiefly concerned with the spatial relations between movements of the fingers made in response to other cognized relations between objects in space (the parts that are being assembled). Consequently, it may be that the 'mechanical' factor[2] extends its influence, beyond the 'mechanical' tests in which it was first observed, to these concrete finger operations. To determine whether this is so we must compare ability at 'routine' assembling with ability at the 'mechanical' tests.

To sum up, theoretical considerations suggest the necessity of comparing together ability at (*a*) various routine assembling operations, (*b*) intelligence tests and (*c*) mechanical aptitude tests, in order to analyse the factors involved in 'routine' assembling, with a view to

[1] Interesting, in this connection, is the statement of one engaged in selecting workers for the assembling room of a very large factory, that she has found the best criterion to be the standard reached on leaving school: but she would nevertheless welcome a better.

[2] I.e. the special group-factor which was found to determine (in part) success at various mechanical aptitude tests devised by the writer. See *op. cit.* p. 5.

arriving at a sound procedure for testing a person's suitability for this kind of work.[1]

5. THE EFFECTS OF 'PRACTICE' AND OF 'TRAINING'.

We have already referred to practice as an influence affecting test scores. In the case of motor tests, the extent to which an individual is likely to improve with practice is of special consideration, since not only is it impossible to obtain a reliable measure of any given motor operation without some repetition of the same movements, but it is usually more important to know how a person will eventually succeed after practising the operation than to measure his ability initially. Hence, an individual's 'improvability' by practice at routine assembling is itself an important object of study, necessitating the practising of subjects in routine assembling operations.

In practice it will usually be impossible and uneconomic to train for any length of time applicants for vocational guidance, or for posts, before testing them. Consequently, it is very important to know how initial ability at the tests compares with ability after more prolonged practice. To throw light on this matter, we must practise subjects at routine operations and compare their final with their initial ability.

Should it turn out that initial ability at a given operation highly correlates with ability after practice, we shall have greatly simplified the task of measurement, since we shall know that those who have been selected on the grounds of their initial performance will at least continue to do well *so far as that operation goes*. But can we conclude that similar improvement will be shown in other operations of the assembling room? Not unless we know that improvability in one operation highly correlates with improvability in others. To decide the latter point our subjects must be practised in more than one operation and comparisons drawn between their improvability in each.

Further indications as to how far a person may ultimately go may be gleaned from the course which improvement takes. A subject who is still progressing is clearly superior to another who, although 'equal' to the former at the moment, has long ceased to improve. Possibly, too, a comparison between the rates and variations[2] of improvement

---

[1] The comparison was also subsequently extended into simple manual tests as described in Chapter VIII.

[2] The function measured by these variations we have called 'variability'.

at different parts of its course may throw interesting light on the question of ultimate ability. These considerations lead to a study of the shapes of the practice curves.

Similar questions arise with respect to 'training' as distinguished in Chapter I from 'practice',[1] and lead to a study of the curve of 'training'. More important, however, where 'training' is concerned, is the study of its wider effects considered in the following paragraphs.

6. The 'transfer' question.

Intimately bound up with the psychology of 'improvability' is the question of transfer. How far does practice in one operation assist when one comes to do another, unpractised, operation? The answer is important both for the light it may throw on the factors involved in assembling work, and for the guidance it would afford in the organization of assembling work within the factory. Workers are frequently transferred from one kind of work to another, and not always on account of necessity. It would be advantageous to know how far fall off in output is likely to result from such changes. Likewise, the suitability of any proposed training scheme can only be satisfactorily judged in relation to the answer to be given to this question. Previous research on the problem has usually been confined to a single, rather restricted, operation differing greatly from the much more complex assembling operations we are concerned with here. It has, therefore, seemed worth while to investigate the problem further. To this end we have compared our subjects' ability at unpractised operations before and after practice at other operations.

As in the case of 'factors', so with 'transfer', it is important to know the breadth over which the latter may extend. For this reason we have secured data on a variety of operations.

Hitherto, in the sphere of manual activities, the problem of 'transfer' has been investigated only with respect to the effects of 'practice'. In the present inquiry we shall extend our examination to the effects of 'training', and develop, for this purpose, a scheme of training based on one of the routine assembling operations.

7. 'Control' subjects.

Should improvement in the unpractised operation be observed, it still remains to be determined whether this may not be due to such

[1] *Supra*, p. 6.

practice as arises from the twice doing of the operation itself,[1] rather than to transfer from a different practised operation. To see whether this is so we must compare such improvement with the performance of a 'control' group who are tested at the unpractised operations under the same conditions as the 'trained' group, but who refrain from the practice undertaken by the trained group.

C. THE MEASUREMENT OF THESE FUNCTIONS

1. ACCURACY.

We have seen that the soundness of our conclusions respecting the relations between the functions we have been considering will depend upon the accuracy with which we may be able to measure the functions themselves. As a check on this we have employed the reliability coefficient[2] wherever possible.

2. THE MEASUREMENT OF 'STATIC' FUNCTIONS.

The intrusion of random errors makes it necessary to repeat a motor performance a certain number of times if we are to secure a reliable measure, even when measuring a static function like 'initial ability'.[3] These repetitions will themselves tend to induce a change of ability on account of practice.[4] Hence our endeavour, in measuring a static function, must be to determine the minimum number of repetitions needed to secure a sufficiently reliable measure.

3. THE MEASUREMENT OF 'DYNAMIC' FUNCTIONS.

Dynamic functions may be measured either 'absolutely' or 'relatively'. Thus we may take as our measure of improvability either the absolute difference between the initial and final abilities, or we may express this difference as a percentage of either of these abilities. The distinction is necessary, since what might apply to (say) a person's absolute improvement might not be true when his initial ability is taken into consideration.

---

[1] I.e. before and after practising the (different) 'practised' operation.
[2] *Supra*, p. 5. [3] *Supra*, p. 18.
[4] Assuming, as is usual, the limit of improvement has not been reached.

D. INTROSPECTIONS, AND OBSERVATIONS
OF INDIVIDUALS

To throw light on the processes involved in assembling, we have ourselves carried out introspections on the various operations and have also received many introspective accounts from our subjects. Moreover, the latter were observed while at work, with a view to discovering individual differences in behaviour which might explain the differences found in the objective measures. Special note was taken of cases which departed widely from the normal.

CHAPTER III

GENERAL PLAN OF RESEARCH

A. OUTLINE OF THE PROGRAMME OF RESEARCH

1. THE BROAD LINES OF INQUIRY.

In the light of the preceding discussion our research has pursued three broad lines of inquiry, viz. (1) that concerned with the nature of and the relations between the abilities measured by 'mechanical' and 'routine' assembling tests; (2) that concerning the psychology of improvement which comes (a) with practice, and (b) with training at 'routine' assembling; and (3) that relating to the question as to whether the effects of (a) practice and (b) training, at one routine assembling operation, transfer to other routine assembling operations. While each of these problems might have provided an ample independent subject of study, they are so inter-related that much was to be gained by collecting data simultaneously from the same subjects respecting all three. This course was also dictated by considerations of economy, since many subjects who were unable to carry out the lengthy practice involved in (2) were able to do the shorter tests required of 'control' subjects in (3), and the data collected for (2) and (3) provided material for investigation (1).

2. PLAN OF COLLECTING DATA.

Before we describe our tests and procedure in detail, it will make for clearness to outline the plan according to which our data have been secured. Briefly, this was as follows:

(a) The same subjects were given tests of 'mechanical' assembling, of 'routine' assembling, of 'mechanical aptitude' and of 'general intelligence'. In addition, such cognate data as those respecting mechanical interests and training, ability at school subjects and ability at drill and games were secured where possible.

(b) Our subjects were then divided into several groups each of which, with one exception, practised daily for a period certain of the routine assembling tests, different operations being practised by different groups. The one exception acted as a 'control' group. It abstained from assembling, or from performing kindred operations, during the period of practice.

(*c*) On completing the practice (or, in the case of 'controls', the period of rest), all subjects were retested on the routine assembling tests.

(*d*) In the 'training' experiments a similar procedure was adopted as in the 'practice' experiments, with the exception that the practice referred to in (*b*) was replaced by a course of training in one of the routine assembling operations (assembling containers). A single 'trained' group thus took the place of the four 'practised' groups of the practice experiments.

3. RANGE OF OPERATIONS.

With a view to extending the range of assembling work investigated, both 'mechanical' and 'routine' tests were so chosen as to include operations widely differing in difficulty and complexity. In the case of 'routine' operations, further differentiation was introduced by including both 'assembling' and 'stripping' operations. In the former, the subject was required to fit together the various pieces provided, while in the latter he was required to take to pieces the object thus assembled.

For similar reasons our subjects underwent practice both at assembling and at stripping; and some (the adult groups) practised one of these double operations, whereas others (the schoolboys) practised two.

4. RANGE OF SUBJECTS.

Conclusions valid with respect to one standard of attainment might not hold with respect to another. In order, therefore, that our inquiry might cover a wide range of ability, data have been secured from adult subjects, from elementary schoolboys, and from elementary schoolgirls, including, in the latter instance, both normal and backward pupils.

Precisely the same programme was not followed in every group. Details of the tests and procedure adopted in the several groups are given later. But both adult and boy groups worked to the same general scheme outlined above. The schoolgirls were prevented by circumstances[1] from carrying out the more prolonged practice involved in

---

[1] The approach of end of term when many left the school.

(*b*) above; so that for these subjects our data were confined to initial ability.[1]

5. TREATMENT OF DATA.

Details will be best given when we examine the data themselves. It may, however, make for clearness to enumerate here more specifically than was desirable in the general discussion of our previous chapter the questions with which we shall be concerned, and the methods we have employed in our attempt to answer them.

(*a*) *The trustworthiness of our measures.* To pursue the inquiries outlined at the beginning of this section presupposed sound measures of the functions which enter into them. Our first concern has, therefore, been to determine, wherever possible, how far these measures agree with themselves as shown by the inter-correlation of two or more attempts to measure the same function. Seldom will such reliability coefficients, as they are termed, indicate perfection in our measures. Their value lies (i) in indicating how far reliability may be increased by a change of procedure in administering the test, and (ii) in insuring that conclusions respecting the relations between different functions are not invalidated through errors of measurement, as indicated by unduly low reliability coefficients.

(*b*) *Influence of practice on reliability.* The reliability coefficient is itself a measure subject to influences which might form an appropriate subject of inquiry in the field of mental measurement. Different methods of measuring reliability may yield different results which in turn may direct attention to the varying influences which have operated in the test. Conversely, where a known variation in the test conditions has occurred, its effect on the reliability coefficient is not without interest, especially when the variation is itself unavoidable in the practical application of the test. Such a variable, in our present data, is the increase in efficiency which results from practice. Here we may distinguish between the short practice involved in a single sitting and the much longer one extending over the special practice period. To investigate the influence of the former we have determined the correlation between the successive performances of the operations which were carried out before the practice period proper, and which constituted our measure of initial ability. To examine the effect of longer

---

[1] I.e. to the measure of ability secured at a single sitting. This itself involved many repetitions of the same operation.

practice on reliability, we have taken the correlations between the successive daily practices which followed these initial performances.

(c) *The relation between static functions.* Having checked the reliability of our measures, we shall proceed to compare these various measures with one another, chiefly by the correlation method, in order to determine how closely they are related. Here we shall deal, first, with what we have called static functions—the abilities measured by the tests—drawing our data principally from the measures of initial ability, since for these our groups are larger, and supplementing this, where possible, by the more exhaustive measures yielded by our practising groups.

The result of this comparison showed a tendency of the various operations to correlate positively with one another. Consequently, our next step was to determine how best to interpret this observed tendency for those who do better at one operation to do better at another. Here our inquiry is concerned with the previously defined 'factors'. We have seen that the test score employed as the measure of ability at the operation tested is usually the resultant of more than one 'influence', and that in the interests of better understanding and measurement we must endeavour to determine what these are, and to measure, in relative isolation, those which we have described as 'factors'.

An example will serve to make clear the main problems in this part of our inquiry. Consider the case where A and B are 'mechanical' assembling tests, C and D are 'routine' assembling tests, and where each test exhibits some degree of positive correlation with each of the others. The questions at issue are: (i) is this observed correlation attributable to a single factor common to all four tests; or, (ii) is the correlation between one pair (say A and B) due to a different factor from that causing the correlation between another pair (such as C and D), and, if so, how are these group-factors arranged; or, (iii) are there both group-factors and a common factor; and (iv), if a common factor is found, is it to be identified with a still wider factor common not only to these assembling tests but also to tests of general intelligence? Should a group-factor be found in the 'mechanical' assembling tests, we shall have the further interesting question as to its relation to the group-factor which previous research has disclosed in our tests of mechanical aptitude.[1] To determine these group-factors we have employed Spearman's tetrad-difference criterion and Yule's theorem of

[1] See J. W. Cox, *Mechanical Aptitude* (London: Methuen and Co. 1928).

partial correlation. Details of our procedure will best be given in our discussion of the results.

(*d*) *The relation between dynamic functions.* We have described as a dynamic function any change which a person's mental trait may undergo. The improvement effected by practice and the subject's variability as shown by irregularities in his curve of practice are the chief dynamic functions entering into the present data. These it will be profitable to compare (i) with one another, (ii) with the subject's general intelligence, and (iii) with his actual ability at the operation. The question as to how best to predict the degree of efficiency to which a person may ultimately attain is of primary importance in this connection.

Our mode of comparing these functions has been that of correlation supplemented by graphs.

(*e*) *The curves of 'practice' and of 'training'.* Equally important in our study of dynamic functions is an examination of the actual daily performance of each subject during the practice period. Such data will be presented in the form of (i) individual practice curves, and (ii) composite practice curves obtained by averaging the daily performance of the whole group. While the former indicate individual differences, the latter serve to emphasize characteristics of the group as a whole. Important differences in these more general features may be disclosed by comparing with one another composite curves for each of the operations practised.

The chief point of interest in the 'training' curves will be the comparison they will afford with the 'practice' curves regarding the rate of progress made under the two conditions.

(*f*) *The transfer of practice effects.* Here our problem is to determine whether practice at one (or more) routine assembling operation tends to increased efficiency in other routine operations. This necessitates (i) testing subjects on a number of operations; (ii) practising some of these subjects at certain of these operations only, while the remainder (the 'control' group) rest; and (iii) re-testing the whole on the unpractised operations. If the practisers do better in (iii) than in (i), it remains to decide whether this is due to the intervening practice at other operations, or merely to the practice which the re-test involved in (iii) necessarily introduces. The answer must be sought by comparing the gain made by the practisers with that of the controls. If the former exceeds the latter, it remains to be determined whether or not such excess may be due to mere chance—the unavoidable variable error. Such determination can only be made by comparing the observed excess with its probable error. Hence, with our larger schoolboy groups we have employed statistical methods.

The adult groups were hardly large enough in some cases to warrant statistical treatment. Results here will be presented graphically. As it happened, the need for statistical treatment proved to be less insistent, since practically no difference between the two groups was found.

In order to afford a safer comparison with those who were trained (on containers), our practisers of the container operation were subsequently increased in number. This allowed of comparison being made between groups of practisers and of controls (and, later on, of trainees) of equal initial ability *at each operation* in which the effects of the practice were sought. Such refinement of technique seems never to have been introduced into previous experiments on 'transfer'. It is rendered desirable by the fact that the effects of a given amount of practice are not the same at different levels of ability. They tend to diminish as one's efficiency increases.[1]

(g) *The transfer of training effects.* In the training experiments we have a similar problem as in the above-mentioned practice experiments; namely, whether the effects of training in one operation (as distinguished from practice) bring about an increase in efficiency in other operations. Our data were examined in the same way as in the practice experiment, both statistically and graphically, and the groups of subjects were large enough to permit of comparisons being made between groups of trainees, of practisers, and of controls of equal initial ability at each operation in respect of which they were compared.

Having attempted this conspectus of our experiment as a whole, we proceed to give details of our tests and subjects, and then to present our results under the several sections into which they fall.

B. DESCRIPTION OF TESTS AND PROCEDURE[2]

1. TESTS OF 'MECHANICAL' ASSEMBLING.

After a careful observation of a large variety of assembling operations in several factories, it was decided to concentrate attention on the operations involved in assembling and wiring an electric lampholder,

---

[1] For further details respecting the relation of practice effects to ability see *infra*, Chapter XII.
[2] Where the name of the test has been abbreviated, the first letter (or two letters) of the name has been used, suffixed in the case of *routine* operations by 'a' (assembling) or 's' (stripping) where confusion might otherwise arise.

for not only do these divide conveniently into three 'mechanical' operations, but the same piece of work, after the method of assembling has been learnt, divides naturally into five 'routine' tests. The 'mechanical' assembling tests were as follows:

(*a*) *Porcelain test* (P). The interior porcelain part of the lampholder, together with its attachments, viz. two metal blocks, two metal pins

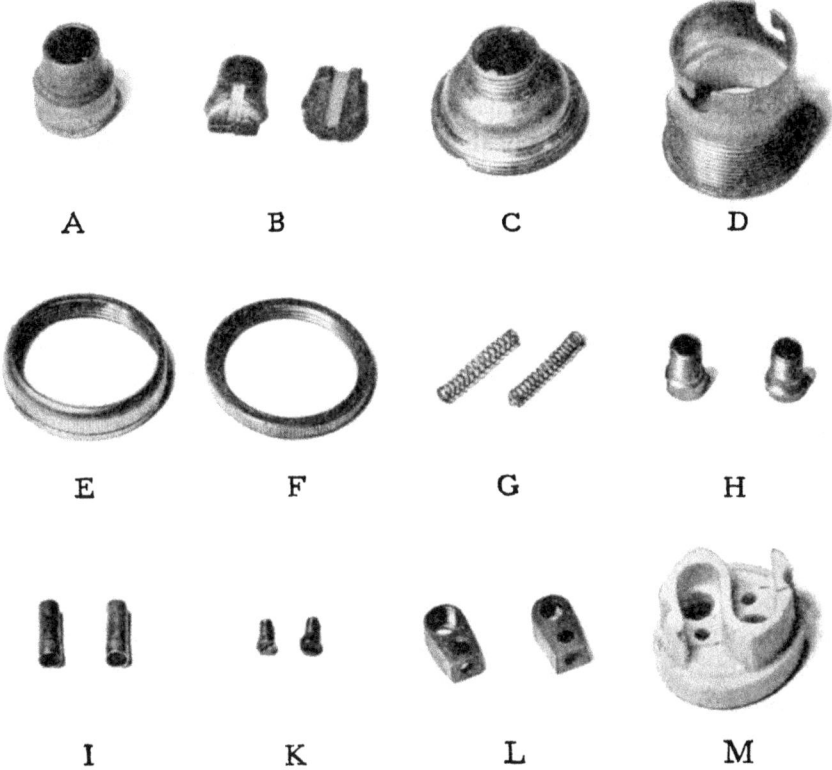

Fig. 1. Parts of the electric lampholder used in the 'mechanical' and the 'routine' assembling operations.

which pass through holes in the blocks, two springs which fit into the pins and two large screws which secure the blocks with the pins and springs to the porcelain part (fig. 1, parts *G–M*).

(*b*) *Container test* (C). The parts of the metal container into which the porcelain part and its attachments fit (fig. 1, parts *A–F*).

(c) *Wiring test* (Wi). This was done after the subject had learnt to assemble (a) and (b). The assembled porcelain part and the separate parts of the container were presented, together with a length of suitably prepared wire and a screwdriver. At one end of the wire was tied a large knot which the subject was told represented the ceiling over which no object could be threaded. The problem was to attach the lamp-holder, properly assembled, to the wire.

PROCEDURE

(a) *Initial ability at 'mechanical' assembling.* In the case of our adult groups,[1] the whole of the parts of both porcelain and container tests were presented together, but in separate rows as shown in fig. 1. The subject was informed that all the parts fitted together to make a single object. He was told that the parts in the bottom row (which formed the 'porcelain' test) could be put together first, and was asked to do this part first if he were able—but if not, to go ahead and assemble as much as he possibly could. He was allowed to give up trying after 15 min. and was given two further trials, each up to 15 min. duration, on subsequent days, after he had promised not to examine a copy of the object in the meantime.[2] If the subject could complete the porcelain part before proceeding to the container, a separate time was secured for each part. Otherwise, only one time could be secured for the two parts. By this procedure most subjects eventually succeeded in assembling the object.

In the case of our elementary school groups, each part was presented separately, viz. parts *A–F* as the 'container' test, and parts *G–M* as the 'porcelain' test. Two trials were allowed at each test. At the porcelain test a third attempt was allowed if needed, and at this last trial an assembled porcelain was also put before the subject. He was permitted to handle this copy but not to take it to pieces. By these means a time score at each test was obtained for almost all our subjects.

The wiring test was given after the subject had first succeeded in assembling both container and porcelain. The elementary schoolboys were allowed a single trial up to 10 min. Most succeeded within this time. Of our adult subjects, the few who needed it were allowed a second trial.

---

[1] Described on p. 36.
[2] All were voluntary subjects who would have no motive for doing so.

Throughout, the subjects were told to work as quickly as possible; at the end of each trial, note was taken of such parts as were correctly assembled if the assembly had not been completed at that sitting. All subjects were questioned and classified, as to their previous knowledge of the material, their mechanical interests and their mechanical knowledge and training. Where the subject was acquainted with either of the operations, the test was not considered or included, as one of 'mechanical' assembling, but he was allowed to do the test in preparation for the routine part.

(*b*) *Transition from 'mechanical' to 'routine' stage.* To throw further light on the processes involved in learning, the above three tests were repeated by our adult subjects, twice in the case of the 'porcelain' and 'container' tests, once in the case of 'wiring'. Each repetition was held on a separate day. Here, as during the initial trials, observational notes were taken down while the subject worked, and introspections were obtained after he had finished the sitting.

2. TESTS OF 'ROUTINE' ASSEMBLING.

This same material was now employed as tests of 'routine' assembling as follows:

(*a*) *Screw test* (S). Ten blocks of the kind shown in fig. 1, *L,* were placed randomly on the left-hand third of a sheet of foolscap placed before the subject, and ten small screws as shown in fig. 1, *K,* were placed upon the right-hand third. The operation consisted in picking up a block and a screw, inserting the latter into the hole of the former, giving it one sharp turn to fix it, and replacing it on the middle third of the foolscap. The time taken to insert ten screws was recorded, and the whole repeated five times.

(*b*) *Porcelain test* (P). Here the time recorded was that taken to assemble parts *M, I, H, L, G* of fig. 1, the whole being repeated five times. The parts were placed before the subject in a shallow cardboard box, divided into five compartments, each containing one kind of part.

(*c*) *Container test* (C). Time taken to assemble parts *C, D, E, F, M,* repeated five times as before.[1]

(*d*) *Wedges test* (We). Time taken to assemble parts *A, B, C,* repeated five times.

[1] It will be observed that the 'container' test used in 'mechanical' assembly included, in addition to these parts, parts *A* and *B*. In this and the following routine assembling tests the material was arranged before the subject in five columns each containing the material or one trial.

(*e*) *Wiring test* (Wi). Time taken to wire five lampholders, the parts constituting the 'porcelain' test, together with the screws *K*, being already assembled.

(*f*) *Stripping tests.* These involved the same material as the above tests (*a*)–(*d*), but the subject was required to take the object to pieces and sort out the parts under standard conditions. Thus, in the 'stripping screw' test, ten blocks with their screws in position were placed in the centre of the foolscap sheet, and the subject was required to undo the screws as quickly as possible, placing the screws on the right-hand third, and the block on the left-hand third, of the paper.

PROCEDURE

(*a*) *Initial ability at 'routine' assembling.* Our adult subjects, after having successfully performed the 'mechanical' assembling operations, were given the above tests (*a*)–(*e*) and, in addition, the 'stripping screw' test which was done at the same time as the 'screw test', in the following manner.

The subject was first timed on inserting ten screws. A few seconds' pause followed while the blocks, with screws now inserted, were arranged randomly in the centre of the paper. The subject then unscrewed them as rapidly as possible. This process was repeated until the whole had been done five times.

In the case of the elementary school subjects, the procedure was modified in the direction of (i) increasing the number of repetitions, and (ii) alternating stripping and assembling in all except the wiring test. Thus fifteen porcelains were assembled in groups of five and alternated with stripping the same porcelains and sorting the parts into the divisions of a box from which they had been taken. 'Wedges' and 'containers' were assembled fifty times in groups of ten, and this alternated with 'stripping' the same parts. 'Wirings' were carried out ten times, each being timed separately.

(*b*) *Practice at 'routine' assembling.*

(1) *Adult group.* After undergoing the tests just described, our adult subjects were divided into four groups, each of which practised one of the operations (*a*)–(*d*), including 'stripping', daily for eleven days, keeping the time of day and general conditions as constant as possible. The daily practice arranged for each operation was as follows:

(α) 'Screwing group.' The daily practice consisted of repeating the screwing test ten times (assembling 100 screws altogether), alternating 'assembling' and 'stripping', in groups of ten, as in the initial 'routine' test. Thus ten records were secured at each sitting for both 'assembling' and 'stripping', each being the time required to assemble (or strip) ten screws.

(β) 'Porcelain group.' Subjects in this group repeated the 'porcelain' routine test four times, assembling twenty 'porcelains' altogether, in groups of five. As with 'screwing', assembling was alternated with 'stripping'.

(γ) 'Container group.' This group repeated the 'container' test eight times daily, assembling forty in all, in groups of five, and alternating the assembling with stripping.

(δ) 'Wedges group.' The 'wedges' test was repeated ten times, making in all fifty repetitions of this operation daily. As before, they were timed in groups of five and alternated with stripping.

Before beginning his period of practice, each subject was presented with a set of typed instructions in which were set out (i) the general conditions under which he was asked to practise; (ii) details relating to the manner of practising the particular operation assigned to him; and (iii) notes for his guidance in making introspective observations.

(2) *Elementary school groups.* Those of our elementary schoolboys who practised were divided into two groups and practised on each of the five school mornings of one week as follows:

Group A practised the 'screws' and 'wedges' tests. In the case of 'screws', eighty were assembled in groups of twenty, and alternated with 'stripping'. Practice at the 'wedges' test consisted of assembling forty wedges in groups of ten, alternating each group with stripping as in the initial routine tests with these subjects.

Group B practised 'porcelains' and 'containers'. The alternate assembling and stripping of five porcelains twice constituted a day's practice. Practice at 'containers' followed the same procedure as for 'wedges', viz. forty assemblings and strippings in alternate groups of ten.

Thus, each group practised four operations, viz. assembling and stripping two objects. Practice always followed the same order, and was confined to mornings only. Each group consisted of twenty subjects and was practised in sections of five, according to a prearranged time-table, so devised that each subject was equally favoured as regards the time at which the practice was taken on the net result of the week's work.[1]

In order to fit the whole of the practice into one morning, it was necessary to practise two sections together. Thus while five of group A practised 'screws', another five practised 'wedges'. The sections would then change over. A section which practised 'screws' first on one morning would practise 'wedges' first on the next morning.

(c) *Terminal ability at 'routine' assembling.* After this period of prolonged practice, each subject was re-tested in all operations as for 'initial' ability.

(d) *Procedure in the 'training' experiment.* In the training experiment the same procedure was followed in the initial and terminal tests as with the adult practice groups. The training, which intervened between these, occupied approximately the same time and was given under the same general conditions as the practice on containers which it replaced. Details respecting the training scheme will be found in Chapter XIII.

Those of our trainees who afterwards *practised* the wedges operation did so under the same conditions as those who practised this operation in the practice experiments.

C. SUBJECTS

1. EXPERIMENTS ON ANALYSIS AND PRACTICE.

(a) *Adult groups.* These were composed of members of the staff of the National Institute of Industrial Psychology, members of the staff of the City of London College and senior students at the College. It included members of both sexes. In our first series of experiments, thirty-three subjects completed the whole programme, including the period of practice, and seventeen acted as 'control' subjects, i.e. they took the initial and final tests, omitting the intervening practice. In a second series, which was carried out in connection with the training experiment, the practisers were increased to thirty-nine and the controls to thirty-one.

In addition, twelve other subjects were able to carry out the practice, but were prevented by circumstances from taking the initial and final tests. Consequently we have been unable to include these in our experiment on 'transfer'. They will, however, provide useful additional data relating to the period of practice itself.

[1] Two members of Group A were unable to complete the entire programme.

(b) *Elementary school groups.*

(i) *Boys.* Thirty-eight boys from the top two classes of an elementary school completed the whole programme of the transfer experiment, i.e. eighteen in group A, twenty in group B. In addition, a further thirty-two completed the initial and final tests as 'controls'. In our subsequent inquiry into the relation of routine assembling tests to simple manual tests, fifty-nine boys of similar educational attainment, but drawn from another school, completed the test programme.

(ii) *Girls.* Three classes of an elementary girls' school were also tested for initial ability at 'screws' and 'wedges', the same procedure being followed as with the boys. They consisted of (a) a backward class of twenty-two pupils specializing in handwork, (b) a fairly bright 'scholarship' class numbering forty-six, and (c) a class of intermediate attainment between these two, numbering thirteen. All were comparable in age with the boys' classes.

Thirty-six of the 'normal' subjects also took the three 'mechanical' assembling tests already described, together with an additional 'gastap' ('mechanical') assembling test, and the remaining 'routine' assembling tests, similar procedure being followed as with the boys.

2. Training experiments.

The subjects for the training experiment were similar in character to those composing the adult groups of our practice experiment. Thirty-six subjects, including members of both sexes, completed the entire programme of initial tests, training (on containers), and terminal re-tests. Thirty-five of these subsequently undertook a period of practice at another operation (wedges).

D. FURTHER DATA COLLECTED

1. Measures of intelligence.

Thirty-eight of our adult group took a comprehensive 'intelligence' test consisting of ten sub-tests, each of 5 min. duration.

Sixty of the boys and all of the girls were given Spearman's "Measure of Intelligence for Schools".

2. Measures of 'mechanical aptitude'.

All of the elementary school subjects took two of the writer's 'mechanical aptitude' tests consisting of ten 'models' (M), and test E 3 (E).[1]

[1] As described by J. W. Cox, *Mechanical Aptitude*, Chapter v (London: Methuen, 1928).

3. STAR PUZZLE AND TAP TESTS.

These were two additional 'mechanical' assembling tests given to some of our elementary school groups. The star-puzzle test required the subject to disengage a star-shaped piece of metal from a pair of metal 'horseshoes'. It was given to all of our schoolboy subjects. The important feature of the test was that, unlike 'mechanical' assembling tests and the usual form of puzzle, it permitted of a second testing in which the subject was required to replace the star on the horseshoes.[1] It thus afforded a means of determining how far such puzzles depend on chance ('trial and error'), since by requiring the subject not only to take the star off but also to put it back, we greatly reduce the chance element.[2]

The tap test (T) was included among the tests given to our schoolgirl groups, with a view to analysing a very simple mechanical assembling test. It consisted in assembling the three simple parts which make a gas tap.

4. SIMPLE MANUAL TESTS.

For the sake of clearness the simple manual tests will be described in Chapter VIII.

5. ABILITY AT SCHOOL SUBJECTS.

The position in class of each of our schoolboys at a recent comprehensive school examination, held just before the tests were given, was secured from the head master, who has co-operated throughout the experiment. Data relating to ability at various school subjects was obtained from the head mistress at the girls' school.

6. ABILITY AT DRILL AND GAMES.

The boys were graded for ability at (*a*) drill and (*b*) games, by the sports master. The time of testing presented a favourable opportunity for securing these, since the school was specially training for the inter-school sports competitions.

7. ESTIMATES OF 'INTELLIGENCE'.

Estimates of 'intelligence' were obtained for those of our adult subjects who were members of the Institute staff from two independent members of the staff to whom they were well known.

---

[1] This required similar knowledge of the relations between the shoes and the star as was involved in taking them apart.

[2] For example, assuming the chance element to be equally operative on each occasion, if of 100 subjects twenty succeed in taking off the star 'by chance', only four (theoretically) should succeed in both taking it off and replacing it 'by chance'.

8. ESTIMATES OF INCENTIVE.

A member of the Institute's staff graded those of our adult group who were known to him according to the general willingness with which they appeared to undertake and carry through the test programme. A similar grading, based on the subject's behaviour while undergoing the test, was made by the writer.

It must not be supposed that any were unwilling subjects. It is, however, conceivable that some were more anxious to excel than others, and that under certain circumstances a lengthy series of tests might become irksome.

In any case such estimates must be treated with caution, for the observations are both difficult to make and difficult to interpret. A person is not prevented from putting forth his best efforts by a preference for some other form of activity. Allowance must be made for the operation of will and intelligence. Moreover, the incentives which operate in the actual test situation must be distinguished from those which may influence general mental attitude towards the test itself. Where effort is to be inferred from the subject's behaviour during the test, the matter is complicated by the facts that (i) effort is itself intimately related to ability—all subjects have not the same energy to expend, however *willing* they may be; (ii) appearances are deceptive, especially in assembly work—the more care one takes to impart accuracy to his movements the less are his fingers apt to move; and (iii) the wise subject soon learns that haste and flurry (which are easily mistaken for endeavour) are detrimental to efficiency, and tries to avoid them.

Notwithstanding these difficulties, it seemed worth while inquiring how far the impressions of two independent assessors might agree and whether they were reflected in the test results.

E. INCENTIVES

The afore-mentioned tests were undergone voluntarily by our adult subjects after the aim and procedure had been fully explained, and their co-operation invited. Consequently, no special incentive was, or could very well have been, offered.

The elementary schoolboys took the tests as part of their school work, after some of the aims of the experiment, and especially its connection with vocational guidance, had been explained. We found the boys very keen to do the tests; so much so that, when selecting individuals for testing, it was difficult throughout to restrain the rest of the class. Subjects were always willing to stay behind after school or during 'play' in order to complete the test which they might happen to be doing. The need for any additional incentive did not, therefore, appear very necessary. Lest, however, the enthusiasm might wane during the period of practice, a small monetary incentive was offered. The boys were told that approximately twenty shillings would be distributed in prizes, which would vary in amount according to the number of points they scored on the whole programme of routine testing, and that these points would depend on (i) their own average times based on the whole performance; (ii) the average times of the sections to which they belonged; (iii) the number of times they beat their best previous times; and (iv) the number of times their section beat its best previous time. In this way both individual competition and group loyalty were appealed to. A sum of twenty-three shillings was afterwards distributed on this basis.[1]

The girls, like the boys, showed evident desire to shine at the tests; and, as circumstances prevented their undertaking the more prolonged period of practice, no monetary incentive was considered necessary. In both schools the atmosphere created by the excellent relations between pupils and staff, and the interest which the latter took in the testing, combined to call forth the best efforts of the pupils, and none who witnessed the tests in progress could doubt the keenness with which both boys and girls applied themselves.

Observations of our adult subjects suggested that a large monetary incentive might even defeat its object by arousing emotional disturbances detrimental to the work. These subjects frequently reported a reduction in speed through 'trying too hard'. Although the *intention* to do one's best was a necessary condition, it seemed better to concentrate on the operation that was being carried out at the moment to the exclusion of thoughts about the 'trying' itself. Analysis indicates that *regulation* and *control* of energy are important factors in motor skill, and that the intrusion of emotionally toned thoughts concerning success or failure are apt to interfere with these.

In both schools a special room was set apart for the testing and every facility was granted for doing the tests under suitable conditions.

---

[1] It was divided approximately equally between practisers and non-practisers, and no member of one group competed with any in the other. Thus all had equal opportunity.

PART II

STATIC FUNCTIONS

CHAPTER IV

RELIABILITY

A. RELIABILITY OF THE MEASURES EMPLOYED

1. ROUTINE TESTS.

(a) *Adults.* (i) *Size of coefficients.* The inter-correlations of the various sub-tests (or 'trials') constituting our routine tests were first calculated for the first thirty-eight adults who took these tests. The average inter-correlation of *one* trial with another, for each test, was as follows: *assembling screws* (10 repetitions = 1 trial), 0·63; *stripping screws* (10 repetitions = 1 trial), 0·66; assembling porcelains (once), 0·38; assembling containers (once), 0·28; assembling wedges (once), 0·18; wiring (once), 0·32. The whole five trials, it will be remembered, were included as the measure of 'initial ability', so that these sub-tests represent but one-fifth of our measure. Thus, in all except the 'screws' test they represent but a single assembling of the object. Notwithstanding the smallness of these samples of performance, all except two coefficients (− 0·07, − 0·05) were positive. This augured well for the combining of these sub-tests into tests, since even these very short trials exhibited some degree of consistency.

With 'porcelains', 'containers', 'wedges' and 'wiring' the consistency of a single trial[1] is, as we should expect, not high. It is clear that in these cases we must attempt to obtain a more exhaustive measure by adding together the five trials—i.e. by combining them into what we have called a 'test'. If we do this,[2] the 'reliability' of the whole test becomes for 'screws in' 0·91, 'screws out' 0·91, 'porce-

---

[1] In these four tests a single trial consists in assembling the object once; in the screw tests it consists in assembling the object ten times.
[2] On the reasonable assumption that a second five trials would correlate on an average as much with one another and with the present five as do the present five with one another.

lains' 0·75, 'containers' 0·70, 'wedges' 0·52, 'wiring' 0·70. Thus, the total of the five trials yields a measure of the performance which possesses a fair degree of consistency with itself.

(ii) *Influence of complexity and number of repetitions.* The trials (sub-tests) at 'screwing', both 'assembling' and 'stripping', are clearly more reliable than those at the other four performances. They differ from the others in two distinct ways, viz. (1) the operations involved are simpler, in the sense that they are fewer in number and are more uniformly carried out both by the same and by different subjects; and (2) they involved ten repetitions, whereas the others involved only one performance. The important question arises, are these observed differences in reliability due to (1) or to (2)? To answer, we must compare the reliability of ten repetitions at these others with the ten repetitions at 'screwing'. Doing so, we find the reliability of the ten trials to be, for 'porcelains' 0·86, 'containers' 0·82, 'wedges' 0·68, and 'wiring' 0·82. On comparing them with the corresponding figures for 'screws', viz. 0·63 and 0·66, it is clear that the apparent lower reliability is wholly accounted for by the fewer repetitions involved in the total 'trial'. Indeed, the more complex tests are, if anything, somewhat more reliable than the simpler ones when they comprise the same number of repetitions.

Important corollary for testing. It follows that 'reliability' depends rather on the number of repetitions than on the complexity of the movements or on the time involved in the operation. If we are to measure a complex motor operation with the same degree of accuracy as a simple one, it is not sufficient to make the tests of equal length; we must ensure that the number of repetitions taken as the measure is about the same in each case. This means that the more complex operation will take longer, as a rule, to measure, and presupposes that due precautions be taken to exclude the intrusion of such vitiating factors as fatigue and boredom which the longer period of testing might otherwise introduce.

(iii) *Practice influences—or random errors?* If we ask why should repetition increase reliability, two possible explanations are suggested, viz. (1) that practice induces more consistency into the subject's actions; or (2) that random errors, such as those due to slight irregularities in the material or in the subject's reactions, tend to be levelled out over successive trials. Examination of the time scores [1] shows that

---

[1] See curves of initial ability, Chapter x, Section C.

the times do, in fact, tend to shorten as the trials proceed. But the coefficients give no indication that the later trials are more reliable than the earlier, and we shall show presently that even the prolonged practice afforded by the 'training' period has a remarkably small influence on the size of the reliability coefficient. The truth would, therefore, seem to rest with the second of these explanations.

That this is so may be readily tested by determining how far the subject's best, second best, third best, etc., performances inter-correlate, instead of taking as we have just done the inter-correlation between his first, second, third, etc., performances. By so doing we reduce the random influences to one-fifth[1]; and, consequently, if our explanation is correct, the correlations should now be larger. If, on the contrary, the 'attenuation' is due to other causes no amount of diminution of random errors will increase the reliability. That a marked increase in the correlations does occur was seen on calculating these inter-correlation coefficients for the four tests where random attenuation seemed greatest. Thus, the average for porcelains now becomes 0·77, for containers 0·69, for wedges 0·56, and for wiring 0·72. They are all very much higher than before. It follows that if we are limited to a single performance, it is better to choose a subject's best, or next best, etc., rather than his first, or second, etc., trial.

The individual coefficients suggest that the best two trials are somewhat more reliable than the others, but the difference is not statistically significant on the basis of the present number of subjects. It would seem that, provided we treat all subjects alike, it matters little, so far as reliability is concerned, which performance we choose,[2] and that usually the best procedure will be to add together all the trials.

(iv) *Practical confirmation of repetition theory.* We saw (p. 42) reasons for believing that if the number of repetitions constituting the measures of the more complex operations were increased to that comprising the simpler and shorter 'screw' tests their reliability should attain at least to that of these latter tests. These reasons were, however, based upon figures derived statistically from the available inter-

---

[1] If for example, on a five-faced die, the faces are numbered 1 to 5 (representing subject's 1st, 2nd, 3rd, etc., *best* performances), the chances are 5 times greater of throwing a 1 out of 5 throws than of throwing a 1 at any given throw.

[2] Except possibly the fifth best (i.e. the worst) trial at 'wedges', where the average inter-correlation with the other trials falls to 0·33.

correlations of the shorter and less exhaustive measures. It remains an interesting question as to how far such prediction would be fulfilled in practice—would the lengthening of the test introduce factors which would diminish its accuracy as a measure and so offset any gain that should, theoretically, follow from such lengthening?

To put this to practical test twenty-two of our adult subjects, none of whom had practised the operation, were given the 'wedges' test under conditions similar to those which originally governed the 'screw' test—the 'wedges' test being chosen as the one of lowest reliability. The number of repetitions was now increased to fifty as follows: the subject first assembled five wedges, then paused while his time was recorded, then assembled a second five; he then stripped five wedges, had his time recorded, and then stripped the second five; this whole cycle was repeated five times in all. He thus alternately assembled and stripped fifty wedges in groups of ten, each ten being divided into two halves by a pause of a few seconds.

The correlation between the total time for the 'odd' groups of ten and that for the 'even' groups proved to be 0·91 and 0·80 for assembling and stripping respectively. On these figures, the correlation of the whole group of fifty repetitions with another similar group becomes 0·95 and 0·89 respectively, as compared with the corresponding 0·91 for each of the 'screw' tests. These figures thus interestingly confirm our theoretical anticipations.

(*b*) *Elementary schoolboys*. (i) *Size of coefficients*. With sixty-eight schoolboys we have computed two measures of reliability, viz. (1) the correlation between the sum of the 'odd' trials and that of the 'even' trials taken at the same test (i.e. 'sitting'); and (2) that between two complete tests taken on different occasions, the occasions being the first and second times the tests were taken. By the latter method the coefficients are: for *assembling*, screws 0·59, wedges 0·39, porcelains 0·32, containers 0·45, wiring 0·60; for *stripping*, screws 0·74, wedges 0·66, porcelains 0·69, containers 0·43. Corresponding figures by the first method will be found in the last paragraph of this chapter in connection with our inquiry into the effects of practice on reliability.

Every coefficient exceeds four and one half times its probable error. Hence, every test has a significant degree of correlation with itself. The coefficients tend to be higher by the first method, which is probably due to the fact that those influences to which we have referred as systematic, both external and internal, tend to change more from one sitting to another[1] than during the same sitting. One such influence is that due to practice. Reference to Table XXXIV indicates that improvement certainly occurs and is most marked where the above-observed difference is greatest, viz. in the 'porcelain' test. Such influence must be clearly distinguished from the practice which occurs within the 'sub-tests' at the same sitting and which tends to be equal when the sum of 'odd' trials is compared with that of 'even' trials. This tendency for the coefficients to be higher by the first method is not attributable to the practice at the other tests which, in the case of the unpractised tests, took place between the two sittings, for similar differences occur in the case of the 'practised' tests, and of the tests taken by the 'control' group where no intervening practice at other tests occurred.

(ii) *Comparison with adult groups.* Direct comparison between the coefficients given above and those already given for adults is not possible, since the tests involve a different number of repetitions. On making allowance for these differences in repetitions, the reliability for the adult subjects is seen to be much the same as that for the schoolboys; thus, the theoretical figure for the same number of repetitions in the adults is for 'porcelain' assembling 0·72, 'containers' 0·82, and 'wedges' 0·68; all of which agree fairly with the corresponding figures given above for schoolboys.

2. 'Intelligence' test and estimates.

(a) *Adults.* The correlation between the sum of the 'odd' sub-tests comprising the 'intelligence' test and that of the 'even' reaches the high figure of 0·92—which means, of course, that the whole test would be expected to exhibit even higher correlation with itself.

(b) *Elementary schoolboys.* The corresponding figure for the test taken by the boys is 0·80. With both groups, then, we have a high degree of consistency in our measures.

(c) *Estimates.* Of our adult group nineteen members only were known to both assessors of intelligence. The correlation between these two estimates was found to be 0·65.

The correlation of the estimates with the intelligence test was 0·55 (nineteen subjects), and 0·43 (twenty-three subjects) respectively. In the latter case, it seemed to the writer that the position on the staff of

---

[1] Especially so as in the case of non-practised tests, and 'control' groups, over a week necessarily intervened between the two sittings.

certain of the subjects might unconsciously influence the assessment. When these, numbering seven, were omitted (their influence on the correlation coefficient being quite unknown when the omission was made), the coefficient rose to 0·53.

The number of subjects is too small for definite conclusions. These figures suggest, however, that the intelligence test measures much the same thing as the estimates, but measures it more thoroughly and consistently, as shown by its higher reliability and its apparent freedom from the unconscious influences noted in the estimate.

3. MECHANICAL APTITUDE TESTS.

(a) *Schoolboys.* The correlation of 'odd' with 'even' sub-tests was for 'models' 0·70, for mechanical 'explanation' (E3) 0·64.

(b) *Schoolgirls.* These tests, designed originally for older subjects and given hitherto only to boys and senior students, were taken by forty-five of our girl subjects. Reliability for 'models', calculated as before, was 0·53, but fell to only 0·16 for E3. Examination of the scores showed that the girls found this test more difficult than did the boys, and that ability within the group was less widely distributed—the scores clustering more closely around the average. This, together with the facts that (1) the number of sub-tests in each of the two parts into which the test was divided for the reliability calculation was small, so that unsuitability in any one would tend to have a relatively large effect on this coefficient, and (2) its mode of presentation possibly appealed less to girls, may account for this fall off in reliability. The correlation of the whole test with 'models' (0·66) suggests (1) as the more likely cause.[1]

4. VARIABILITY.

Reference to the curves of practice shows that, although all subjects improve as practice continues, the curve of practice is by no means smooth. We have measured the extent to which irregularities occur by determining for each day the amount by which the day's performance deviates from the average of the three days of which it is the middle one, and summing these deviations. This value we have called the subjects' 'variability'. The extent to which such a value is a consistent measure of a definite trait is shown by the correlation of the

[1] It is important to distinguish between the correlation of 0·66—satisfactory as a *reference value* in the present research—and that required for the satisfactory measurement of 'mechanical aptitude' itself. For this a whole team of tests would be needed.

sum of the deviations on the 'odd' days of practice with those on the 'even' days. These were as follows: *assembling*, screws 0·86, wedges 0·50, porcelains 0·63, containers 0·63; *stripping*, screws 0·55, wedges 0·63, porcelains 0·69, containers 0·50. Owing to the limited number of subjects in our adult practised groups, much importance cannot be attached to the actual sizes of the figures; but they serve to show that 'variability' is not a mere 'chance' effect, but a definite trait susceptible to measurement.

5. INCENTIVE.

The correlation between the two estimates of 'incentive' obtained for our adult group was 0·65. Whether or not these estimates measure what they purport to measure, there was evidently something in common between the impressions made on the minds of the assessors with respect to this trait. We have taken as our measure the average of the two assessments.

B. INFLUENCE OF PRACTICE ON RELIABILITY

1. TWO DISTINCT QUESTIONS.

We have now considered the 'reliability' of the chief measures that enter into our data and have seen that, although their 'consistency' as thus indicated is not perfect—which, in view of the complexity of the operations measured, we should hardly expect—there is fair, and in some cases very high, agreement within the measures themselves. Such coefficients serve the even more important purpose of helping us to interpret the correlations which may be found to exist between these different measures.

There remains to consider another important question, especially where the measurement of 'motor' operations is concerned, namely, how will the reliability of a measurement be affected by the degree of practice the subjects may have had at the operations measured? For example, will a test which has been found highly reliable when applied to relatively unpractised individuals remain so when applied to persons who have had longer training? This question must be clearly distinguished from another with which it is apt to be confused, namely, how does ability 'initially' compare with ability at a later stage of practice? It would not, of course, be a reliable procedure to measure an unpractised group against a practised group—not necessarily because the measures (tests) are themselves intrinsically bad, but because we should be measuring two different things. This concerns the influence of practice on ability; at present we are concerned with its influence on 'reliability'.

2. ADULTS.

In order to investigate the question, the reliability of each of the tests practised by our adult groups was determined on each day of practice. Examination of the resulting eleven coefficients, thus obtained for each test, indicated that notwithstanding the considerable progress made during this period, as shown by the practice curves of Chapter x, this had no effect on the reliability of the test. Thus, for assembling screws the reliability is 0·98 on the first day, 0·98 on the last (i.e. eleventh), 1·00 (the highest) on the second, 0·81 (the lowest) on the fifth, and fluctuates irregularly between these limits over the other days. For assembling containers, which showed least reliability, the figures are, 0·69 (first day), 0·50 (eleventh and last day), the highest 0·86 on the ninth and tenth days, the lowest 0·50 on the eighth and eleventh days, and the other coefficients fluctuate between these limits. The coefficients of the remaining six operations lead to the same conclusion, that during the period of eleven daily practices with which we are here concerned, the practice had no effect on the reliability of the daily measure of ability.

All of the coefficients were high, seventy-two out of the total eighty-eight exceed 0·8, forty-eight of these exceed 0·9. Although the groups are too small (9—13 subjects) to attach much importance to the size of any one coefficient, they all point to the same conclusion, and agree with the larger groups of elementary schoolboys.

3. ELEMENTARY SCHOOLBOYS.

In the case of the schoolboys the reliability of the scores was calculated for the first, third and fifth (i.e. last) days of practice. For the twenty who practised 'screws' and 'wedges' the figures for the three successive days were: *assembling*, screws 0·63, 0·77, 0·61, wedges 0·76, 0·77, 0·81; *stripping*, screws 0·82, 0·82, 0·84, wedges 0·91, 0·79, 0·88. Similar figures for 'porcelains' and 'containers' were obtained from the second group. They thus confirm the conclusions arrived at with our adult groups.

CHAPTER V

THE RELATIONS BETWEEN STATIC FUNCTIONS

A. INFLUENCE OF KNOWLEDGE AND INTEREST ON 'MECHANICAL' ASSEMBLING

Like most material ordinarily used in this type of assembling test, the electric lampholder is a commercial object, accessible to and used by the public. Consequently, some of our adult subjects were already acquainted with it—or parts of it[1]—before being tested. This detracted from its efficacy as a measure of 'mechanical' assembling in these cases. Our chief purpose in giving the test to this group was to ensure that all knew clearly how to assemble the parts of the object before employing them as tests of 'routine' assembling, and to secure introspections. Since divergences with respect to previous knowledge of the material so clearly existed, it seemed worth while to inquire into its effect on the test results, and, at the same time, to see how far a general interest in mechanical things might influence the scores at mechanical assembling, even when previous specific knowledge of the test material itself is absent.

For this purpose our subjects were divided as follows: group I had some previous knowledge concerning the mode of assemblage and had mechanical interests; group II had similar previous knowledge but were uninterested in mechanical things; group III had no such previous knowledge but had mechanical interests; group IV had neither previous knowledge nor mechanical interests.

Examination of the times of each group indicates the great advantage which comes, as we should expect, from some previous acquaintance with the material, especially when combined with mechanical interest.[2] Where the latter is lacking, the initial advantage derived from previous acquaintance with the material is less evident. In the container test these subjects do much better initially than either of the groups where previous knowledge is lacking; but they number

[1] More particularly the 'container' part which had been employed as a test at the Institute.
[2] Tables and graphs of these data may be seen at the National Institute of Industrial Psychology. It has been found too costly to print all the tables and graphs that will be referred to in this book.

only two. Where the times for completely assembling the lampholder are concerned, they are actually surpassed by those who started with no prior knowledge but were interested in mechanical things. Here, too, so far as it goes, interest proved a better criterion of success than knowledge where interest was lacking.[1]

Perhaps the most interesting feature brought out by the data is the significant rôle played by interest. In all three operations, where subjects start equal as regards knowledge of the object, those with mechanical interests do much better than the others. This advantage which seems to derive from interest in other mechanical things (the groups are not large enough to provide conclusive evidence) does not mean, necessarily, that knowledge of these latter has 'transferred' to the present test. In view of the general narrowness of transfer of this kind, a more likely explanation would seem to be that the interest itself is largely the result of the same natural aptitude which enables the subject to shine at the tests.

B. MECHANICAL TESTS COMPARED WITH ONE ANOTHER AND WITH 'INTELLIGENCE'

1. SCHOOLBOYS.

Having seen that our measures were sufficiently reliable to ensure that any lack of correlation between them could not arise from inconsistency in the measures themselves, our next step was to inquire how far they measured the same thing, as shown by the correlation between them. In view of the considerations of the preceding section, we confined this part of our inquiry to our school groups, for of these subjects none of the girls and very few of the boys had met with the material before.[2]

Table I gives the inter-correlations of the tests of 'mechanical' assembling, mechanical aptitude and intelligence. From these the influence of such slight correlation as was found with 'age' has been eliminated by Yule's formula for partial correlation, although the resulting changes in the coefficients were inappreciable.

[1] Such lack of any general interest in mechanical objects must, of course, be distinguished from lack of interest in the test. Here all subjects, so far as we could observe, endeavoured to do their best.

[2] The children were questioned before they knew that they were to be asked to assemble the object, and under these conditions they were anxious to claim more knowledge, rather than less. The one or two boys who had some previous acquaintance with the parts of a lampholder were excluded.

The following conclusions emerge from the table:

(1) Each mechanical assembling test measures something in common with each of the other two, as shown by its positive correlation with them.

(2) Similarly as regards the mechanical aptitude tests.

Table I.

Inter-correlation of 'mechanical' assembling, mechanical aptitude, and intelligence data. Age eliminated. Sixty schoolboys. (Decimal points omitted.)

		C	P	Wi	E	M	I	Ex	Age	'g'
Mechanical assembling	C	—	38	24	25	29	08	14	24	13
			A			**B**		**C**		
	P	38	—	36	51	55	38	33	25	42
	Wi	24	36	—	57	35	13	29	15	23
Mechanical aptitude	E	25	51	57	—	72	30	36	01	39
			F			**E**		**D**		
	M	29	55	35	72	—	28	32	04	36
Intelligence	I	08	38	13	30	28	—	71	05	[84]
	Ex	14	33	29	36	32	71	—	–01	—
	Age	24	25	15	01	04	05	–01	—	—
	'g'	13	42	23	39	36	[84]	—	—	—

Coefficients over 0·30 exceed 4 times the probable error. 'g' = general factor.

AVERAGES.

A = 0·33 ('mechanical' assembling).
E = 0·72 (mechanical aptitude).
A, B, E, F = 0·42 (assembling and aptitude).
Assembling *v.* aptitude = 0·42.
Assembling *v.* 'intelligence' = 0·23.
Assembling *v.* 'g' = 0·26.
Aptitude *v.* 'intelligence' = 0·32.
Aptitude *v.* 'g' = 0·38.
Assembling and aptitude *v.* 'intelligence' = 0·26.

(3) The general intelligence test correlates highly with the comprehensive school examination, so that both measure very much in common.

(4) The mechanical assembling tests measure something in common with the aptitude tests, as shown by the coefficients in square B, and are possibly somewhat more closely related to these than to one another.

(5) The mechanical aptitude tests are more closely related to one another than to the assembling tests, and also than are the assembling tests to one another.

(6) Both the assembling and the aptitude tests are related to the intelligence test and to the school examination, but much less closely than are the latter pair to one another.

(7) The mechanical aptitude tests are more closely related to each other than to either the intelligence test or the examination.

(8) Similarly as regards the assembling tests, but the difference is less marked.

2. SCHOOLGIRLS.

Similar data from our girl subjects, given in Table II, point to the same general conclusions. The average inter-correlation of the assembling tests, both with each other and with the intelligence tests, agrees very closely with the corresponding figures for the boys. The somewhat lower correlation between the aptitude tests is possibly due to their lower reliability in this group. An alternative explanation may lie in their higher correlation with the intelligence test, suggesting that with girls general intelligence plays a relatively greater part, and the 'mechanical' factor[1] a relatively smaller part. But before attaching much importance to this observed difference, further corroboration is desirable.

The results, viewed as a whole, suggest that success at the mechanical group of tests (i.e. mechanical assembling and mechanical aptitude tests) depends on (1) a factor which they share in common with the intelligence group, and (2) a factor (or factors) peculiar to themselves. The latter is more clearly evidenced in the higher inter-correlation of the aptitude tests, where, indeed, previous research had already indicated a special or 'group' factor of this kind. It becomes, therefore, especially pertinent to ask how far the present data confirm this result, and whether the assembling tests likewise depend on a group-factor. If so, the further question arises as to whether such a factor is to be identified with that of the mechanical aptitude tests. The possibility of additional group-factors must also be considered.

The replies to these questions depend on the above-observed relations and differences between the correlation coefficients. Hence no

[1] Previous research indicates that success at the mechanical aptitude tests depends on these two factors—a result corroborated in the present work.

answer can be given with any degree of certainty until it is known whether these differences are sufficient to warrant the belief that they may have arisen otherwise than by mere chance. For this purpose we need a statistical criterion for determining how far such observed differences may rightly be taken to signify a definite cause (factor), and

Table II.

Inter-correlation of 'mechanical' assembling, mechanical aptitude, and intelligence data. Age eliminated. Thirty-six schoolgirls. (Decimal points omitted.)

		C	P	Wi	T	E	M	I(o.)	I(e.)	Age	'g'
Mechanical assembling	C	—	40	42	22	45	38	43	25	06	37
	P	40	—	34	24	50	65	51	31	-10	44
	Wi	42	34	—	37	27	52	15	04	22	12
	T	22	24	37	—	04	23	27	01	51	06
Mechanical aptitude	E	45	50	27	04	—	59	50	49	07	55
	M	38	65	52	23	59	—	43	37	-10	44
Intelligence	I (odd)	43	51	15	27	50	43	—	80	20	[89]
	I (even)	25	31	04	01	49	37	80	—	11	—
	Age	06	-10	22	51	07	-10	20	11	—	—
	'g'	37	44	12	06	55	44	[89]	—	—	—

(Labels within table: A and B and C in P row area; F, E, D in E row area.)

'g' = general factor.

AVERAGES.

A = 0·33 (assembling), omitting T = 0·39.
E = 0·59 (aptitude).
A, B, E, F = 0·37.
Assembling v. aptitude = 0·38.
Assembling v. 'intelligence' = 0·25.
Assembling v. 'g' = 0·25.
Aptitude v. 'intelligence' = 0·45.
Aptitude v. 'g' = 0·50.

how far, on the contrary, they may be merely the fluctuations which we expect in all statistical data, and which, in the present instance, have their origin in the probable errors of the correlation coefficients. The application of such a criterion is reserved for a later section in order that the relations between other parts of our data may first be examined.

3. STAR PUZZLE TEST.

Table III gives the inter-correlations of that remaining member of our test group which we have classed, broadly, as 'mechanical', namely the puzzle test. It will be remembered that in this test the subject was required first to discover how to take off a star-shaped piece of metal from a pair of horseshoe-shaped pieces between which it was held by chains connecting the two horseshoes, and then to replace it. The 'significant' correlation of 0·43 between these two performances indicates that the 'taking off' is not wholly a matter of chance, or of 'trial and error'.

Table III.

Inter-correlation of puzzle test with 'mechanical' assembling and other data. Sixty schoolboys. (Decimal points omitted.)

	C	P	Wi	Puzzle off	Puzzle on	Puzzle off and on	E	M	I
Puzzle off	−03	28	10	—	43	82	22	28	14
Puzzle on	−04	04	05	43	—	78	14	24	10
Puzzle off and on	01	22	09	82	78	—	16	18	11

The correlation of 'puzzle off' with the assembling tests is with one exception (the rather complex porcelain test) negligible. It is somewhat higher with the aptitude tests; but is much lower, here, than are the assembling tests themselves—facts which suggest it to be, in the light of our subsequent analysis, less suited to the measurement of mechanical ability. The correlation with 'intelligence' is interesting. It, as also the higher correlation with the aptitude tests, is in conformity with our analytical results.

C. 'ROUTINE' ASSEMBLING TESTS COMPARED WITH ONE ANOTHER AND WITH 'INTELLIGENCE' AND 'INCENTIVE'

1. ADULTS.

Table IV gives the inter-correlations of the 'initial' tests at the six operations carried out by thirty-three of our adult group. The general tendency is towards a positive inter-correlation, which in many cases exceeds four times the probable error. In the case of 'porcelains', 'containers', 'wedges' and 'wiring' the inter-correlations are, however, sometimes negligibly small. We saw in the last chapter that the individual trials constituting these tests are not, taken singly, very 're-liable', and have suggested the influence of random errors as an explanation. We have also noticed that a marked increase of correlation results from reducing this influence. If we apply this same reason-

Table IV.

Inter-correlation of 'routine' operations as measured by total 'initial' trials. Thirty-three adults. (Decimal points omitted.)

	S_a	S_s	P_a	C_a	We_a	Wi
S_a	—	59	50	37	07	25
S_s	59	—	37	19	13	−06
P_a	50	37	—	56	22	51
C_a	37	19	56	—	16	60
We_a	07	13	22	16	—	31
Wi	25	−06	51	60	31	—

ing to the inter-correlations of the different operations by selecting, as our measure, the best of the five trials rather than their sum, we should hardly expect a generally higher correlation, because our measure is not now so 'saturated' with the function it attempts to measure. On the other hand, it seems reasonable to expect more uniformity in the resulting table, since the variable influences in the measures will have been reduced. The results of so doing are given in Table V,

Table V.

Inter-correlation of six routine operations as measured by the best of five trials. Thirty-nine adults. (Decimal points omitted.)

	S_a	S_s	P_a	C_a	We_a	Wi
S_a	—	45	44	40	25	20
S_s	45	—	19	20	13	40
P_a	44	19	—	37	40	35
C_a	40	20	37	—	19	23
We_a	25	13	40	19	—	20
Wi	20	40	35	23	20	—

where this greater uniformity does make its appearance. A comparison of the table suggests that with more reliable means of measuring them a much higher positive correlation might be found to run throughout these operations.

If we turn to a more reliable measure, viz. the total ability of the subject as measured by the whole practice period, we do indeed find a marked positive correlation. But here we are limited to few subjects and to only two, in some respects similar, operations, viz. 'assembling' and 'stripping' the same material. Further confirmation, however, is found in the inter-correlations of total ability at the more diverse operations practised by our somewhat larger schoolboy groups (cf. Tables VII and VIII).

Table VI gives the correlations of the comprehensive test of intelligence, and of the combined estimate of 'incentive', with the six routine operations. Clearly, from these figures, the observed inter-correlations of the routine tests cannot be ascribed to the operation of 'intelligence' or of 'incentive'. For explanation we must look, rather, for something peculiar, or, to use a technical expression, 'specific', to the tests themselves.

Table VI.

Inter-correlation of 'routine' assembling operations with 'intelligence' test and 'incentive' estimate. Adult group. (Decimal points omitted.)

	S_a	S_s	P_a	C_a	We_a	Wi	Int.	No. of S
Intelligence	−13	−09	−32	−16	−02	−16	—	42
Incentive	−07	08	25	17	14	12	10	36

The figures for the 'porcelain' test are interesting as suggesting that 'incentive' may have played a small part here—it was the longest and most difficult of the tests. If so, its negative correlation with 'intelligence' may, perhaps, be explained by supposing that those who held the more responsible posts on the staff (and who, generally speaking, did better at the 'intelligence' test) had less incentive to give a good account of themselves at the 'routine' test. They were also more inclined to regard themselves as clumsy with their fingers—a view which may have acted adversely on their work. Possibly, however, the figures call for no explanation at all (except 'chance'!), for both are well below four times the value of the probable error.

2. SCHOOLBOYS.

(a) *Initial measures.* The data from the elementary schoolboys (Table VII) lead to similar results as were reached with the adults. The inter-correlations of the assembling operations are in every case positive. Their average inter-correlation (0·35) closely approximates to that for the adult group (0·33). They are, however, like the corresponding figures for the girls' groups, more uniform in size. This may

Table VII.

Inter-correlation of routine assembling tests, examinations and intelligence. Sixty elementary schoolboys. Age eliminated. (Decimal points omitted.)

		S	We	P	C	Wi	S	We	P	C	I	Ex	Age	'g'
Assembling	S	—	33	38	49	30	28	26	33	12	28	31	06	35
	We	33	—	45	30	42	18	39	22	25	07	21	-22	14
	P	38	45	—	26	30	16	22	29	14	22	24	27	27
	C	49	30	26	—	29	-05	33	-02	31	16	28	04	25
	Wi	30	42	30	29	—	23	31	37	21	16	11	08	16
Stripping	S	28	18	16	-05	23	—	31	30	05	23	16	04	23
	We	26	39	22	33	31	31	—	06	49	08	07	17	09
	P	33	22	29	-02	37	30	06	—	15	29	22	23	30
	C	12	25	14	31	21	05	49	15	—	25	12	16	20
Intelligence	I	28	07	22	16	16	23	08	29	25	—	71	05	[84]
	Ex	31	21	24	28	11	16	07	22	12	71	—	-01	—

(Labels in table: A between We/P assembling; B in stripping-S/We assembling area; C near Intelligence; D in stripping; E in stripping)

AVERAGES.

A=0·35.　B=0·28.　C=0·20.　D=0·23.　E=0·18.
Assembling v. 'g'=0·23.　　　Stripping v. 'g'=0·15.

be due to the more exhaustive nature of the tests as given to these groups, involving, as they did, many more repetitions of the operation.

The inter-correlations of the 'stripping' operations are also positive, but lower as a group (average 0·23) than for 'assembling'. There are also larger divergences in size, three of the six coefficients being negligible, while the other three are comparable in size with the inter-correlation of the assembling tests.

With two exceptions the inter-correlations of 'assembling' with 'stripping' (rectangle B) are likewise positive. The average value (0·28) is intermediate in size between that for 'assembling' (square A) and that for 'stripping' (square D). While many of the coefficients closely approximate to this average value, divergences approximating to zero occur in some instances. On the whole, however, they exhibit more uniformity than those for 'stripping', but less than those for 'assembling'.

It is further seen that both 'assembling' and 'stripping' tests tend to correlate positively with the two measures of 'intelligence', namely the intelligence test and the comprehensive school examination, but to a less extent than they do with one another. Some of the figures are of negligible size when considered in relation to the number of subjects. A similar (low) correlation with 'intelligence' is, however, observable in the corresponding data from the girls' groups.

(*b*) *Total ability*. For those of our subjects who carried out the five daily practices we have a still more exhaustive measure of ability in the total time taken to effect the whole of this work. The inter-correlations of these measures of the total ability are given in Table VIII.

Table VIII.

Routine assembling. Inter-correlation of total ability at five daily practices. Schoolboys. (Decimal points omitted.)

| | | Group B. Twenty subjects | | | | | | Group A. Sixteen subjects | | | | |
| | | Assembling | | Stripping | | | | Assembling | | Stripping | | |
		S	We	S	We	I		P	C	P	C	I
Assembling	S	—	59	22	32	07	P	—	85	49	57	36
	We	59	—	18	49	−11	C	85	—	37	56	10
Stripping	S	22	18	—	45	52	P	49	37	—	15	54
	We	32	49	45	—	14	C	57	56	15	—	31
	I	07	−11	52	14	—	I	36	10	54	31	—

In every case the figures are positive, and in nearly every instance they are higher than the corresponding figures in Table VII. This is particularly noticeable in the 'assembling' operations which now reach figures (0·59 and 0·85) well over six times their probable errors. It suggests, again, that with this added comprehensiveness our measures have become more 'saturated' with the quality (or qualities) upon which success at the operations depends.

For such operations as are included, the same general characteristics of Table VII reappear, viz. a higher inter-correlation for 'assembling' operations than for 'stripping', and greater variation in the coefficients when confined to the latter (cf. 0·45, the correlation between stripping screws and stripping wedges, with 0·15, that between stripping porcelains and stripping containers). The small size of the groups makes it necessary to accept these figures with caution; but their broad indication of a positive relationship between the routine operations, which tends to be closer in the 'assembling' group, thus far confirms the results of Table VII.

The same general relation with the 'intelligence' test as was observed in our measures of 'initial' ability reappears in these more exhaustive measures of 'total' ability. The tendency is, again, towards positive correlation—in some instances fairly high, but in others of negligible amount. Now, however, the coefficients are highest for the less complex, 'stripping', operations, whereas the converse is the case for our 'initial' measures, both for the boys already examined and for several girls' groups yet to be considered. This result, taken in conjunction with the previously noted tendency for the correlation between the more complex operations to increase as our measures of them become more exhaustive, conforms with the view that the factor (or factors) introduced in these operations is something other than that measured by the 'intelligence' test.

3. SCHOOLGIRLS.

(a) *'Normal' groups*. Similar results are seen in Table IX which gives, for our girl subjects, data comparable with those of Table VII. Again, the operations tend towards positive inter-correlation, are more marked for 'assembling', and less uniform for 'stripping'; and again there is a tendency towards positive and lower correlation with 'intelligence'.

Four of the operations, measured precisely as before (for 'initial' ability), were carried out by a larger group of fifty-nine girls. For these, suitable records of ability at school subjects were also available. They were pooled into (a) an English group, (b) a handwork group (principally needlework and drawing) and (c) the remaining school subjects. The correlations are given in Table X. The routine opera-

Table IX.

Routine assembling. Age eliminated. Thirty-six schoolgirls.
(Decimal points omitted.)

		S	We	P	C	Wi	S	We	P	C	I(o.)	I(e.)	Age	'g'
Assembling	S	—	55	14	23	43	02	25	26	-08	31	11	46	21
	We	55	—	44	35	58	15	32	12	-13	38	18	39	29
	P	14	44	— (A)	49	55	03	28	32	17	31	27	37	32
	C	23	35	49	—	43	40	25	47	07	18	21	35	22
	Wi	43	58	55	43	—	31	40	25	05	49	42	27	51
Stripping	S	02	15	03	40	31	—	06	35	-21	29	42	51	39
	We	25	32	28	25	40	06	—	10	16	13	00	55	00
	P	26	12	32	47	25	35	10	—	38	11	01	18	04
	C	-08	-13	17	07	05	-21	16	38	—	14	00	60	00
Intelligence	I (odd)	31	38	31	18	49	29	13	11	14	—	80	20	[89]
	I (even)	11	18	27	21	42	42	00	01	00	80	—	11	—

(Quadrant labels B, C, D, E marked within the table.)

AVERAGES.

A = 0·42.   B = 0·20.   C = 0·29.   D = 0·14.   E = 0·18.
Assembling *v.* 'g' = 0·31.   Stripping *v.* 'g' = 0·11.

tions again manifest the same general relations to one another as were observed in the earlier tables, as do their low correlations with the intelligence tests. Their only appreciable correlation with the subjects of the school curriculum occurs with the handwork group—and here it falls to zero where the simplest operation (stripping screws) is concerned. The school subjects, on the other hand, all exhibit some correlation with one another and with 'intelligence'—in this respect agreeing with the data of Table VII (boys).

A comparison of the four quarters into which the table is divided thus *suggests* the presence of a factor in the routine operations distinguishable from that in the intelligence test and school subjects. Both factors appear in handwork.

(*b*) *Backward group.* (i) *Measurement.* We have seen that in our adult subjects there was little to choose between the successive repetitions of the operation on the score of reliability, and that the sum of all the repetitions afforded the best measure—a practice which we have followed with the more exhaustive measures of 'initial' ability secured from our normal school groups. It seemed not unlikely, however, that our backward girls might be slower in understanding the general requirements of the test, and that this might be reflected in the first trial (the sum of ten repetitions) making it less reliable than the four trials which followed and completed our measure of 'initial' ability. If so, the sum of the last four trials would provide a better measure for this group than would the sum of all five trials. To test this we determined

Table X.

Routine assembling, intelligence and school subjects. Age eliminated. Fifty-nine girls. (Decimal points omitted.)

		S	We	S	We	I	English	Other subjects	Hand-work
Assembling	S	—	50	23	23	13	15	−11	20
	We	50	—	18	54	15	08	−07	38
Stripping	S	23	18	—	29	02	12	11	−05
	We	23	54	29	—	06	−01	−04	29
	I	13	15	02	06	[74]	35	18	27
English		15	08	12	−01	35	—	23	39
Other subjects		−11	−07	11	−04	18	23	—	23
Handwork		20	38	−05	29	27	39	23	—

AVERAGES.

Routine *v.* routine = 0·33.   Routine *v.* school subjects = 0·03.
Routine *v.* intelligence = 0·09.   Routine *v.* handwork = 0·21.

the inter-correlations of the various tests which result from taking as measures (1) the sum of the five trials, (2) the sum of the last four trials and (3) the first trials.

The inter-correlations based on (2) as the measure (which average 0·54) were in every case higher than those based on (1) (average 0·39), while those based on (3) were, without exception, lower still (average 0·15). In this group we have, therefore, treated the first trial as a learning period, and have taken the sum of the remaining four trials as our measure in the work which follows.

Correlations of the first trials with the 'intelligence' test proved to be, for assembling screws − 0·03, assembling wedges 0·30, stripping screws 0·14 and stripping wedges 0·06. It is clear that, with the possible exception of 'assembling' wedges, whatever factor may have intruded into these first trials, it can hardly have been 'intelligence'. The figure for 'assembling wedges' is interesting in that this operation was the only one where the subject was required to follow simple instructions about handling the materials—a fact which probably accounts for its relatively high value in the first trial, and its fall off to 0·18 in subsequent trials (see Table XI).

Although this group is too small, by itself, to allow of definite conclusions, it may be remarked that the three types of measure noted above are in complete accord with what has already been said about the tendency for the various tests to draw closer together as they become more reliable and exhaustive.

(ii) *Inter-correlation.* In Table XI we have, for our comparable group of backward girls, data similar to that derived from our normal

Table XI.

Routine assembling compared with intelligence and school subjects. Age eliminated. Twenty-two backward girls. (Decimal points omitted.)

		S	We	S	We	I	English	Arithmetic	Handwork	Age
Assembling	S	—	70	51	46	10	−03	00	22	01
	We	70	—	53	60	18	16	13	40	08
Stripping	S	51	53	—	48	09	02	03	17	32
	We	46	60	48	—	−08	00	−01	00	20
I		10	18	09	−08	[66]	64	22	21	43
English		−03	16	02	00	64	—	10	46	49
Arithmetic		00	13	03	−01	22	10	—	11	39
Handwork		22	40	17	00	21	46	11	—	59

AVERAGES.

Routine *v.* routine = 0·55.   Routine *v.* school subjects = 0·04.
Routine *v.* intelligence = 0·07.   Routine *v.* handwork = 0·20.

groups. The number of subjects was necessarily restricted to the size of the class—twenty-two—and ability at arithmetic had to be substituted for the 'other subjects' of Table X. The degree of mental retardation may be gauged from their average score at the intelligence test (93·7) as compared with that for our group of fifty-nine 'normal' girls (115·2)—figures in which the close correspondence between progress in school and ability at the test is again indicated, and which suggest, incidentally, that the more general employment of such tests as aids in grading and in predicting ability in schools is long overdue.

The positive inter-correlation of the routine assembling operations again appears and reaches the high average of 0·55. The figure for 'assembling' operations (0·70) is, as hitherto, higher than that for 'stripping' (0·48).

In every instance the figures are higher than the corresponding ones for our normal group—that for 'stripping' now closely approximates to the coefficient for 'assembling' with the normals. In view of the size of the groups, too much importance must not be placed on the actual size of these figures, but, taken in the aggregate, they support the view that the mentally backward find the operations more complex —a suggestion borne out by their longer times shown in Table XXXIII.

The inter-correlations of the intelligence test and school subjects again prove to be positive in every case (lower right-hand quarter of the table), whereas, with the exception of handwork, their correlation with the routine operations approaches zero. Handwork again correlates with both groups of data, and to about the same extent as was observed with our normal group: and the previously noted tendency for this correlation to be somewhat higher with the more complex processes is once more evident. The whole table thus shows a remarkable correspondence with the same data for normal groups and suggests that the relations here observed may hold for a wide range of ability.

D. 'MECHANICAL' TESTS COMPARED WITH 'ROUTINE' TESTS

Without making any implication at this stage as to the unitary factors which may underlie our tests, we have, for convenience of reference, classified these tests into (a) a 'mechanical' group (mechanical assembling and mechanical aptitude), (b) a 'routine' group (routine assembling and stripping), and (c) an 'intelligence' group (general intelligence test and school subjects). We have seen that, in general, the members of these three groups have more in common with members of their own group than with members of another group. We have also noticed that the relative sizes of the correlation coefficients are such as to suggest a group-factor (or factors) in (a) and in (b), i.e. that the ability measured by the members of each of these groups is not wholly the same as that measured by the 'intelligence' group—always provided that these observations are statistically significant.

So far, however, we have seen nothing to show how the ability involved in the (*a*) operations may be related to that in the (*b*) group. Both 'mechanical' assembling and 'routine' assembling involve manual activity. Both the mechanical aptitude tests and the routine assembling operations (especially the more complex) involve the arranging of material spatially. Moreover, both groups tend to correlate with the 'intelligence' group. To find a positive relationship between the 'mechanical' and the 'routine' groups would, therefore, hardly be surprising. The important question then would be to decide how far such relationship might be accounted for by the correlation which the two groups exhibit in common with 'intelligence', and how far by factors peculiar to members of the two groups.

The relevant data are given in Tables XII and XIII. Unfortunately we are here limited to the two groups that took all of the necessary

Table XII.

'Routine' assembling compared with 'mechanical' assembling, mechanical aptitude and intelligence. Age eliminated. Sixty schoolboys. (Decimal points omitted.)

		Routine										
		Assembling					Stripping					
		S	We	P	C	Wi	S	We	P	C	I	Ex
Mechanical assembling	C	25	20	31	15	12	19	09	19	14	08	14
	P	29	17	30	24	34	10	07	17	21	38	33
	Wi	11	04	28	16	19	01	24	03	16	16	29
Mechanical aptitude	E	42	28	42	29	47	15	28	26	15	30	36
	M	40	26	39	27	39	18	15	15	00	28	32
Intelligence	I	28	07	22	16	16	23	08	29	25	—	71
	Ex	31	21	24	28	11	16	07	22	12	71	—

(Section labels within table: P, Q, A; R, S, B; C, D, E.)

AVERAGES.

P = 0·21.   A = 0·23.
Q = 0·13.   B = 0·32.
R = 0·36.   C = 0·20.
S = 0·17.   D = 0·18.

tests, viz. our sixty schoolboys and thirty-six schoolgirls. The evidence provided by each table is, however, strengthened by the close correspondence which exists between the two. The following observations apply to both tables:

Comparing first the 'mechanical' group with the 'routine' group, we notice (1) a positive correlation between the 'mechanical' group and 'routine' assembling tests (rectangles P and R), (2) a much lower,

Table XIII.

'Routine' assembling compared with 'mechanical' assembling, mechanical aptitude and intelligence. Age eliminated. Thirty-six schoolgirls. (Decimal points omitted.)

| | | Routine | | | | | | | | | | |
| | | Assembling | | | | Stripping | | | | | |
		S	We	P	C	Wi	S	We	P	C	I(o.)	I(e.)
Mechanical assembling	C	36	30	27	17	33	36	23	27	–16	42	26
	P	30	49	30	16	38	–04	27	04	–08	49	30
	Wi	45	52	13	17	40	13	–04	15	–12	18	06
	T	31	41	34	19	58	–03	42	12	–05	33	07
Mechanical aptitude	E	35	28	18	24	28	18	01	07	07	50	49
	M	25	40	28	18	45	15	17	–02	04	42	37
Intelligence	I (odd)	31	38	31	18	49	29	13	11	14	—	80
	I (even)	11	18	27	21	42	42	00	01	00	80	—

(Rectangle labels: P under Assembling/P–C of row P; Q under Stripping of row P; R under Assembling of row E; S under Stripping of row E; C under Assembling of I(odd); D under Stripping of I(odd); A at I(o.)/I(e.) of row P; B at I(o.)/I(e.) of row E; E at I(o.)/I(e.) of I(odd))

AVERAGES.

P = 0·33.   A = 0·26.
Q = 0·09.   B = 0·45.
R = 0·29.   C = 0·29.
S = 0·08.   D = 0·18.

and frequently zero, correlation between the mechanical group and 'stripping' (rectangles Q and S).

Comparing, now, these two with the 'intelligence' group, it will be seen that the latter correlates with them to about the same extent as they correlate with one another. Thus, the average inter-correlation of 'mechanical' assembling with 'routine' assembling (boys) is 0·21, while that of each of these with 'intelligence' is 0·23 and 0·20 respectively. Again, the figure for 'mechanical' assembling *versus* 'stripping' is 0·13, while 'stripping' *versus* 'intelligence' is 0·18. Similarly, mechanical aptitude correlates with 'routine' assembling and stripping 0·36 and 0·17 respectively, while its correlation with 'intelligence' is 0·32. Like results emerge from the girls' data (Table XIII). It is, therefore, not unlikely that the correlations observed here may be wholly accounted for by a single factor common to all three groups. There is certainly not the same clear suggestion of group-factors in these inter-correlations of 'mechanical' with 'routine' tests as was observed in the inter-correlations of these tests with themselves.

At the same time, the average values of certain of the rectangles (in particular R of Table XII and P of Table XIII) are slightly in excess of the theoretical value required on the basis of a single factor running throughout the table; and differences in magnitude occur both in the individual coefficients and in the groups (cf. the average of P with that of R in Table XII). The importance to be attached to these differences will depend on the probable errors of the coefficients in which they are observed. The application of the criterion for determining what statistical significance they may possess will be found in our next chapter.

E. SUMMARY

The chief results discussed in this chapter may be summarized as follows:

1. Previous knowledge and training are apt to vitiate measures of 'mechanical' assembling which involve the use of common objects, and must be carefully guarded against.

2. Interest and ability in mechanical operations tend to go together.

3. Mechanical assembling and mechanical aptitude tests have much in common with one another.

4. 'Intelligence' and school subjects have much in common.

5. 'Routine' assembling operations have much in common, especially where fairly complex in character.

6. Measures of different 'routine' operations exhibit closer relationship as they become more exhaustive.

7. Except in adult subjects (where further evidence is desirable), 'mechanical' tests and 'routine' tests exhibit some relationship with 'intelligence', which is rather closer in the former than in the latter group of tests.

8. This relation is less close than that exhibited by the members of each group of tests with one another.

9. The 'mechanical' tests exhibit some relation with the 'routine' tests, though hardly more than might be accounted for by their common correlation with 'intelligence'.

10. Handwork is the only member of the 'subjects' group showing any appreciable correlation with routine assembling. It also correlates to about the same extent with 'intelligence' and with other school subjects.

11. 'Incentive' (as and where estimated) played little part in determining the relationships between the routine operations.

12. Special (or group) factors are suggested in (*a*) the 'mechanical' tests and (*b*) the 'routine' tests. These need the employment of a statistical criterion for their complete determination.

CHAPTER VI

THE FACTORS IN 'MECHANICAL' ASSEMBLING

A. ULTIMATE ANALYSIS

1. Necessity and implication of ultimate analysis.

Even when highly reliable tests have been secured and these exhibit high positive inter-correlation, we should seriously err if we were to conclude that this correlation was itself a sufficient proof of the existence of a unitary special ability which determined success at these tests and which was measured directly by the test scores. Before any conclusion respecting a special ability can be drawn, it must first be determined how far the observed correlation may be attributed to a *general* ability, i.e. to one which extends its influence over the whole (or a wider) range of mental tests. Even should it prove otherwise, we are still left with the question as to the range of the special ability and whether it functions in unitary fashion.

In brief, we must push our analysis beyond the concrete products of the mental activity, as measured by the test score taken at its face value, into the mental causes, or influences, which determine the score. In accord with our definitions,[1] the end-products of such analysis will be 'mental factors', and the test score (purified of random and systematic errors) will be their 'function'. Such analysis into ultimate factors is, of course, solely concerned with the way in which the mind functions when performing various operations. It throws no light on the subjective nature of the factors.

Knowledge of these factors is of more than theoretical interest. They provide the 'abilities' into which alone all vocations, occupations, jobs —indeed any human task—can be profitably analysed, for only entities which function in unitary fashion can be measured; and we cannot hope to predict, with any degree of precision, ability at an occupation from known ability at mental tests unless both are analysed in terms of the same unitary factors.

---

[1] See p. 17.

2. THE CRITERION ADOPTED.

Let the inter-correlation of four tests, a, b, p and q, be denoted by r_{ap}, r_{aq}, r_{bp} and r_{bq}. Consider, first, the case where the only factor common to any pair of the tests is one common to all four. Then some positive correlation would be expected between each pair of tests on account of this common factor. Its magnitude would depend upon the extent to which success at each of the pairs in question depends on this factor (i.e. were 'saturated' with it) as compared with a factor *specific* (or peculiar) to the individual tests. Suppose a and p were highly saturated with the factor, while in b and q it entered to only a small extent. We should then expect r_{ap} to be high and r_{bq} to be low; and further, r_{aq} and r_{bp} to be of intermediate magnitude, since in each of these cases the saturation is high in one test and low in the other. More strictly, it has been shown that theoretically the product of r_{aq} and r_{bp} will equal the product of r_{ap} and r_{bq}; and, conversely, when these products are equal the correlations are necessarily attributable to one and the same factor.[1] This condition for a single common factor may be more conveniently expressed as $r_{ap}.r_{bq} - r_{aq}.r_{bp}$ (known as the tetrad difference, and denoted by F) = 0.

In practice, each correlation coefficient contains a 'sampling' error; consequently so does the tetrad difference (F). Hence, even when this condition holds theoretically, the experimental value of F will tend to be some small positive or negative value rather than zero itself. Only when this value exceeds that to be expected from chance or accidental circumstances can the condition be regarded as not satisfied.[2] This will be determined by its 'sampling' (or probable) error.[3]

If the condition holds for more than four tests the experimental values of the F's of all the possible tetrads, divided in each case by its probable error, will tend to distribute normally around zero in agreement with the law of error. This, then, will be the criterion for a single factor common to a large group of tests.

3. THE CASE OF A GROUP-FACTOR.

Consider, now, the case where $r_{ap}.r_{bq}$ is definitely larger than $r_{aq}.r_{bp}$. This will occur when either (or possibly both) of the former pair is too large in comparison with the others to be accounted for

---

[1] C. Spearman, *Proc. Roy. Soc.* A, 1922, cı, 97–100.

[2] I.e. when the tetrad difference exceeds about $4\frac{1}{2}$ times its probable error.

[3] For calculating this we have employed formula 15 of C. Spearman, *The Abilities of Man*, Appendix, p. xi.

wholly by the same factor. The cause of this super-correlation must be sought in some factor (or factors) common to the pair of tests in which it occurs. Similar remarks apply to r_{aq} and r_{bp}, when their product exceeds $r_{ap} \cdot r_{bq}$.

Since F here tends to some significant value, it is clear that the F's derived from a group of such tetrads will no longer conform to normality of distribution. Consequently, this tendency for the F's to scatter more widely on either side of zero than could be attributed to chance will provide the criterion for a factor common to only certain pairs of tests, i.e. for a group-factor.

The precise location of this factor in the tetrad must be sought in an analysis of the data. If we have reason for supposing a group-factor in certain tests, the tetrads may be so arranged that the correlation between pairs of these is always a factor in the left-hand product. The F's of these *directed* tetrads will then, if our supposition is correct, distribute around some significant positive value.

4. METHOD OF APPLYING CRITERION.

In the present research we have employed directed tetrads of the kind $r_{t_1 t_2} \cdot r_{ei} - r_{t_1 i} \cdot r_{e t_2} = F$, where t_1, t_2 are any two tests (e.g. the assembling operations) to be examined for a group-factor, and e, i are two comprehensive measures of general intelligence. The group-factor will be indicated by the tendency of F to be positive and 'significant'. Its location in t_1, t_2 rather than in e, i will be dictated by the analysis of the tests, and by the unreasonableness (in the light of this analysis and of previous research) of assuming the only alternative, namely, that the assembling operations (t_1, t_2) are better measures of intelligence than are the school examinations and the general intelligence tests (e, i).

B. FURTHER EVIDENCE OF THE 'MECHANICAL' FACTOR IN MECHANICAL APTITUDE TESTS

To test for a group-factor in the mechanical aptitude tests, we must examine tetrads of the kind

$$F = r_{m_1 m_2} \cdot r_{i_2 i_1} - r_{m_1 i_1} \cdot r_{i_2 m_2},$$

where m_1, m_2 are the mechanical aptitude tests, and i_1, i_2 are measures of 'intelligence'.[1] Two tetrads of this kind are available from the boys'

---

[1] In the boys' data the measures of intelligence are the general intelligence test and the comprehensive school examination; in the girls' data they are the two halves of the intelligence test.

data (Table I) and two from the girls' (Table II). The values of F in the former are 0·4152 and 0·4104 with a p.e. 0·0554; in the latter, 0·2613 and 0·2870 with a p.e. 0·066. The figures for the boys, being well over 7 times the probable error, clearly indicate the presence of a group-factor and thus confirm our previous results.[1] Of the figures for the girls, one is very nearly 4 times, the other is 4·35 times, the probable error. While less conclusive than those for the boys, they strongly suggest that the group-factor is also operative in the case of the girls. This conclusion is strengthened by the finding of a similar factor in the girls' scores at 'mechanical' assembling.

C. A GROUP-FACTOR IN 'MECHANICAL' ASSEMBLING

Consider, now, tetrads of the type

$$F = r_{a_1 a_2} \cdot r_{i_2 i_1} - r_{a_1 i_1} \cdot r_{i_2 a_2},$$

where a_1, a_2 are any two mechanical assembling tests, and i_1, i_2 the two measures of intelligence as before. The distribution of such F's (divided by their probable errors) taken from Tables I and II are given in Table XIV.

Table XIV.

Mid-value F/p.e.	+ 1·5	2·5	3·5	4·5	5·5	6·5
Frequency, Boys	—	—	3	0	2	1
Frequency, Girls	2	4	2	4	—	—

The F's are in every case positive and, on the combined result, scatter around approximately 3·6 times the probable error instead of the zero to be expected if the correlation were due to the same factor throughout. Here, then, is evidence of a group-factor (or factors) in the mechanical assembling tests.

Is there, we may further ask, a group-factor common to the assembling and the aptitude tests? To determine this we must examine tetrads of the type

$$F = r_{a m_1} \cdot r_{i m_2} - r_{a m_2} \cdot r_{i m_1},$$

where a, m, and i signify, as previously, assembling, aptitude and intelligence tests, respectively. Here one of the assembling tests of our last tetrad is replaced by one of the aptitude tests (i.e. rectangle B replaces rectangle A of Tables I and II). Their distribution, given in Table XV, now provides evidence of a group-factor (or factors)

---

[1] Described in the writer's *Mechanical Aptitude* (Methuen and Co. 1928).

common to mechanical assembling and mechanical aptitude tests. Tetrad differences well over $4\frac{1}{2}$ times the probable error are found with both sexes. The approximate central values around which the F's are equally distributed are seen to deviate from the zero expected by

Table XV.

Mid-value F/p.e.	1·5	−0·5	+0·5	1·5	2·5	3·5	4·5	5·5	6·5	7·5
Frequency, Boys	—	—	—	—	1	4	2	3	1	1
Frequency, Girls	1	—	1	1	7	2	0	3	1	—

chance—markedly so in the case of the boys. The only negative value occurs in the case of test T (the gas tap), where success depends more upon manipulative skill than on ability to solve the very simple problem which it presents; and where, consequently, we should not expect a 'mechanical' factor to have much influence.

D. IDENTIFICATION OF THE THREE GROUP-FACTORS AS A SINGLE 'MECHANICAL' FACTOR

1. CORRELATION WITH THE MORE GENERAL FACTOR.

The evidence so far examined indicates the presence of a group-factor (or factors) common to the mechanical aptitude tests, one (or more) common to the mechanical assembling tests, and one (or more) common to both classes of test.[1] We have now to inquire whether these factors are to be identified as one and the same factor.

At first sight it might seem sufficient for this purpose to apply the criterion for a single factor to the inter-correlations of these tests. But this procedure would overlook the fact that the tests all show a tendency—in some cases quite high—to correlate with the measures of intelligence. Consequently, we must conclude that, over and above such group-factors as our evidence may disclose as 'special' to these assembling and aptitude tests, there exists another factor of wider generality which extends its influence beyond these tests into the intelligence measures and causes their observed correlation with intelligence. Accordingly, the influence of this wider factor must be removed before the relations between the group-factors can be examined.

To this end, we have calculated the correlation of each test with this

[1] For reasons for locating the factors in these rather than in the 'intelligence' measures see p. 70.

more general factor.[1] The resulting coefficients are given in the last column of Tables I and II.

2. SPECIFIC CORRELATION.

We may now employ these coefficients, in conjunction with Yule's theorem for partial correlation, to determine the correlation remaining

Table XVI.

Specific correlation, i.e. influence of the general factor eliminated from Table I. Mechanical assembling and mechanical aptitude tests. Sixty boys. (Decimal points omitted.)

		C	P	Wi	E	M	'*m*'
Assembling	C	—	36	22	22	26	39
	P	36	A —	30	41	B 47	63
	Wi	22	30	—	54	30	51
Aptitude	E	22	41	54	—	68	80
	M	26	47	30	68	—	71

AVERAGES.

A = 0·29.   B = 0·37.

Table XVII.

Specific correlation, i.e. influence of the general factor eliminated from Table II. Mechanical assembling and mechanical aptitude tests. Thirty-six girls. (Decimal points omitted.)

		C	P	Wi	T	E	M	'*m*'
Assembling	C	—	29	41	17	32	26	51
	P	29	—	32	19	35	57	63
	Wi	41	32	A —	36	25	B 52	71
	T	17	19	36	—	-07	18	25
Aptitude	E	32	35	25	-07	—	46	43
	M	26	57	52	18	46	—	77

AVERAGES.

A = 0·29.   B = 0·30.

---

[1] 'General' in the sense that it is common to all the tests in the table, as shown by their inter-correlations. The method employed is described by Spearman (in reference to '*g*') in *The Abilities of Man*, p. xvi. While our results are in general accord with Spearman's theory of '*g*', it should be noted that neither the statistical methods, nor the present interpretation of the observed correlations, *presuppose* any theory of mental relationships.

after the influence of this general factor has been removed. These residual (or 'specific') correlations are given in Tables XVI and XVII. The application of the tetrad–difference criterion has already led us to expect some specific correlation on account of the group-factor. These tables indicate the extent to which such correlation actually occurs. Except for the rather higher figure for the aptitude tests with boys, the figures show general agreement for both sexes.

3. APPLICATION OF THE CRITERION.

In these specific correlations we have the data for determining the relations between the previously observed group-factors, for we may now apply the criterion for a single factor to these. Doing so, we get the following distribution of F:

Table XVIII.

	(+ and −)		
Mid-value F/p.e.	0·5	1·5	2·5
Frequency, Boys	7	3	5
Frequency, Girls	11	8	1

In no instance can F be regarded as of statistical significance, for nowhere does it reach even 3 times the probable error. Consequently, nowhere in these tables of specific correlations is there evidence of any factor other than the single (group) factor to which they must all be attributed. The three group-factors disclosed in Sections B and C thus prove to be one and the same 'mechanical' factor common to the assembling and the aptitude tests.

E. OBJECTIVE ANALYSIS OF 'MECHANICAL' ASSEMBLING

1. RESOLUTION INTO MEASURABLE 'ABILITIES'.

In our last chapter a crude comparison of the correlation coefficients suggested that, although the mechanical assembling and the aptitude tests had something in common with the intelligence tests, they had more in common with one another. The present analysis has indicated that this closer relation seen in the coefficients is not without statistical significance; moreover, that it can be wholly explained by a single factor running throughout the mechanical group of tests. Seeing that the correlations are far short of unity, we must suppose that the score at each test is also partly conditioned by a further influence which is peculiar (or 'specific') to each particular test. This specific part may be something intrinsic to, and inseparable from, the mental operations involved in the test; or it may be merely an accidental circumstance intruding, as an error, into the measurement. Since, by nature, the specific factors vary from one test to another, they will tend to cancel one another in a team of 'mechanical' tests. The measurable 'abilities', then, which have any degree of generality in our data, are (*a*) a special ability (or factor) common to the mechanical tests, and (*b*) a more general ability common both to these and to the measures of general intelligence.

Since the mechanical assembling tests involve, in addition to a mechanical problem, the practical manipulation of the parts into position, the question arises as to whether this manipulative activity introduces a group-factor. This question is considered in the analyses which follow; but we may anticipate our conclusions by saying that they suggest that the activity enters largely *specifically*, i.e. as a different factor in each test, and so accounts, at least in part, for the specific part of the test score.

2. DEGREE OF 'SATURATION'.

The analysis also affords a means of giving more precise determination to these factors, for the specific correlations may now be employed to calculate how far each test correlates with the group-factor.[1] Hence there may be compared the respective merits of the tests as measures of the factor. These figures are given in the last column of Tables XVI and XVII. They indicate that (1) the aptitude tests are more highly 'saturated' with the group-factor than are the assembling tests;[2] and (2) in the assembling tests the saturation tends to increase with the difficulty of the test. Thus they provide valuable guidance in the choice and construction of tests for measuring this special factor.

By comparing these correlations with those for the general factor (last columns of Tables I and II), it is seen (1) that with one exception[3] the tests are more dependent on the mechanical factor than on the general factor; and (2) that this dependence on the mechanical factor as compared with the general factor is greater in the mechanical aptitude tests.

[1] By methods similar to those employed for determining the correlation with the general factor. These are described in the writer's *Mechanical Aptitude*, p. 205.
[2] With the exception of the 'explanation' test (E) when given to the girls' group. We have already noticed its lower reliability with this group.
[3] See footnote 2 above.

The last observation is based on our larger boys' group. In the case of the girls' group, an exception occurs in the case of the 'wiring' test; and there is a general tendency for the assembling tests to exhibit more correlation with the mechanical factor than they show in the boys. It is possible that previous 'mechanical' experience plays some part in the boys' results in this kind of test and so tends to lessen its value as a measure of innate mechanical aptitude. At the same time, too much importance must not be assigned to the actual magnitude of the correlations obtained from the girls' group alone, owing to its small size.

3. COROLLARY FOR MEASUREMENT.

It follows, as a corollary, that a team of suitable mechanical aptitude tests may be expected to yield a better measure of the mechanical factor than a team of mechanical assembling tests.[1] This does not mean that tests of the assembling type may not find useful application when testing for a specific task which is known to involve both mechanical understanding and practical manipulation. But here, it must be remembered, we have no evidence that the assembling tests do in fact involve this manipulative part as a *group-factor*, and, consequently, as a *measurable ability*. On the contrary, the analyses we have yet to examine suggest that it functions as a different *specific* factor in each test, and that, in any case, the *routine* assembling tests provide a better measure of any general underlying manipulative ability. Consequently, a more scientific and accurate procedure would be to analyse the occupation in terms of the mechanical and the manipulative factors and to measure these separately.

[1] See also p. 236.

CHAPTER VII

FACTORS IN 'ROUTINE' ASSEMBLING

A. EVIDENCE OF A GROUP-FACTOR IN THE 'ROUTINE' ASSEMBLING TESTS

1. NORMAL BOYS AND GIRLS.

We have next to consider, in relation to the routine tests, questions similar to those raised in the last chapter about the mechanical assembling tests; in particular, how far is there evidence of *special* ability in the routine operations, and is this best conceived as a unitary ability running throughout these operations, or as a number of independent abilities? The relevant tetrads are of the kind

$$r_{R_1 R_2} \cdot r_{i_2 i_1} - r_{R_1 i_1} \cdot r_{R_2 i_2} = F,$$

where the R's denote any two routine tests and the i's are, as before, two measures of general intelligence. The routine tests divide into two kinds, viz. 'assembling' and 'stripping'. Consequently they yield three classes of tetrads:

(1) where the R's are both 'assembling' tests,
(2) where they are both 'stripping' tests, and
(3) where one is 'assembling' and the other 'stripping'.

For analytical purposes the three classes have been kept separate. Their distributions for our normal school pupils are given in Tables XIX, XX and XXI, the 'direction' of the tetrads being, as before, that given in the above formula.

With few exceptions the F's are seen to be positive and to centre round a value which departs, in many cases, markedly from zero. Here again, then, is evidence both of a group-factor (or factors) and of its presence in the results of both sexes.

The departure from zero is greater where the routine tests in the tetrad are both of the 'assembling' type (compare the first rows of Tables XIX–XXI with the others). This confirms the suggestion which arose previously when comparing the correlation coefficients—that the part played by the factor tends to be larger in the 'assembling' than in the 'stripping' operations.

The fact that the F/p.e. values tend to be smaller in Table XX is due, in part, to the larger probable error consequent on the smaller size of this group. For our larger girls' group (Table XXI), we have included the English mark as an additional reference value for 'intelligence'.

Table XIX. Sixty schoolboys.

Mid-value F/p.e.	− 2·5	1·5	0·5	+ 0·5	1·5	2·5	3·5	4·5	5·5	6·5	7·5	8·5	Central value (approx.)
Both r's 'assembling'	—	—	—	—	—	—	2	9	3	3	3	—	4·9 p.e.
Both r's 'stripping'	—	—	1	3	2	0	0	2	2	0	0	2	3·0 p.e.
One 'assembling', one 'stripping'	2	2	0	2	5	2	15	3	7	2	—	—	3·5 p.e.
Total...	2	2	1	5	7	2	17	14	12	5	3	2	4·0 p.e.

Table XX. Thirty-six schoolgirls.

Mid-value F/p.e.	− 3·5	2·5	1·5	0·5	+ 0·5	1·5	2·5	3·5	4·5	5·5	6·5	Central value (approx.)
Both r's 'assembling'	—	—	—	—	1	2	1	2	6	5	3	4·7 p.e.
Both r's 'stripping'	1	1	0	1	1	2	2	1	1	2	—	2·0 p.e.
One 'assembling', one 'stripping'	—	—	3	7	4	5	4	9	5	2	1	2·3 p.e.
Total...	1	1	3	8	6	9	7	12	12	9	4	3·1 p.e.

Table XXI. Fifty-nine schoolgirls.

Mid-value F/p.e.	+ 1·5	2·5	3·5	4·5	5·5	6·5	7·5
Both r's 'assembling'	—	—	1	1	0	1	—
Both r's 'stripping'	—	2	0	1	—	—	—
One 'assembling', one 'stripping'	4	3	2	2	0	0	1
Total...	4	5	3	4	0	1	1

In those tetrads where the more reliable 'intelligence' test is alone employed for this purpose, the tetrad differences tend to be still higher —two are (approx.) 3·5 times the probable error and the rest are 2·5, 4·5, 6·5 and 7·5 times respectively—but here we are limited to six tetrads.

2. Backward girls.

While evidence from so small a class as our backward girls must needs carry little weight by itself, its consideration in conjunction with the foregoing results seems not unprofitable. We have, therefore, computed the tetrad differences of Table XI, taking as our reference values for intelligence the correlations of the intelligence test with itself and with English. All are positive; of the available eighteen, five are (approx.) 4·5 times, twelve 3·5 times, and one is 2·5 times the probable error. The indication of the group-factor thus extends into the data from this backward group. As before, the tetrad differences are somewhat larger where the 'assembling' operations (as contrasted with 'stripping') are concerned.

B. UNITARY NATURE OF THE 'ROUTINE' ASSEMBLING FACTOR

1. SPECIFIC CORRELATION.

There now arises the same problem as was previously considered in relation to the 'mechanical' assembling tests—does the super-correlation observed between certain pairs of routine tests provide evidence of more than one group-factor, or is it explained by the same factor operating throughout? To put the question in practical form, if we

Table XXII.

Specific correlation. Influence of the general factor eliminated from Table VII. Routine assembling. Sixty boys. (Decimal points omitted.)

		Assembling					Stripping				
		S	We	P	C	Wi	S	We	P	C	'Ma'
Assembling	S	—	30	32	44	26	22	24	25	05	56
	We	30	—	43	28	41	15	38	19	23	65
	P	32	43	— (A)	21	27	10	20 (B)	23	09	48
	C	44	28	21	—	26	-11	32	-10	27	37
	Wi	26	41	27	26	—	20	30	35	18	61
Stripping	S	22	15	10	-11	20	—	30	25	00	26
	We	24	38	20	32	30	30	— (C)	03	48	61
	P	25	19	23	-10	35	25	03	—	09	32
	C	05	23	09	27	18	00	48	09	—	33

'Ma' = routine manual factor.

AVERAGES.

A = 0·32.   B = 0·19.   C = 0·19.
'Assembling' v. routine factor = 0·53.
'Stripping' v. routine factor = 0·38.

wish to estimate a person's success at the kind of work covered by the routine assembling operations, are we to measure one, or a number, of *special* abilities?

As before, the problem is complicated by the correlation with the intelligence tests—a fact which renders it necessary to eliminate this

Table XXIII.

Routine assembling. Specific correlations, i.e. influence of the general factor eliminated from Table IX. Thirty-six schoolgirls. (Decimal points omitted.)

		Assembling					Stripping			
		S	We	P	C	Wi	S	We	P	C
Assembling	S	—	53	07	20	39	07	26	26	−08
	We	53	—	39	31	53	03	34	11	−14
	P	07	39	— A	46	48	−11	30 B	34	18
	C	20	31	46	—	38	35	26	48	06
	Wi	39	53	48	38	—	13	46	27	06
Stripping	S	07	03	−11	35	13	—	07	36	−23
	We	26	34	30	26	46	07	—	10	16
	P	26	11	34 D	48	27	36	10 C	—	38
	C	−08	−14	18	06	06	−23	16	38	—

AVERAGES.

A = 0·37.   B = 0·18.   C = 0·14.

general influence of 'intelligence' before the relations between the group-factors can be determined. We have, therefore, calculated, on the basis of their correlations with the measures of 'intelligence', the correlation of each 'routine' test with this wider factor which they evidently share in common with the intelligence tests, and have then employed these correlations to determine the magnitude of the corre-lation after the influence of this factor has been eliminated.[1] The corre-lations with the factor general to the whole table are given in the last columns of Tables VII and IX, and the specific correlations which result on its removal are given in Tables XXII and XXIII.

[1] By the same method as was employed with the 'mechanical' assembling data. (See p. 73.)

2. APPLICATION OF CRITERION.

(a) *Boys.* The coefficients of these latter tables indicate the magnitude of the correlation attributable to the group-factor, or factors, which the analysis of Tables VII and IX has disclosed. These may now be examined by the tetrad-difference criterion to determine how far they may be accounted for by one and the same factor. The data yield five different kinds of tetrad according to the way in which the 'assembling' and the 'stripping' tests enter into it. Particulars of their distribution and magnitude for Table XXII (boys) are given in Table XXIV, where the a's signify 'assembling' tests, the s's 'stripping' tests and the F's are always taken in the direction shown in the formula.

Table XXIV. Sixty schoolboys.

Mid-value F/p.e.	3.5	2.5	1.5	$\overset{-}{0.5}$	$\overset{+}{0.5}$	1.5	2.5	3.5	4.5
1. $F=r_{a_1a_2}\cdot r_{s_1s_2}-r_{a_1s_2}\cdot r_{s_1a_2}$	1	2	19	21	27	23	14	10	3
2. $F=r_{a_1a_3}\cdot r_{a_2a_4}-r_{a_1a_4}\cdot r_{a_2a_3}$	1	2	1	4	5	1	1	—	—
3. $F=r_{s_1s_3}\cdot r_{s_2s_4}-r_{s_1s_4}\cdot r_{s_2s_3}$	—	1	0	0	1	0	1	—	—

4. $F=r_{a_1a_2}\cdot r_{s_1a_3}-r_{a_1a_3}\cdot r_{s_1a_2}$ 2 at 3·5 p.e., 15 at 2·5 p.e., remaining 103 < 2 p.e.

5. $F=r_{s_1a_1}\cdot r_{s_3s_2}-r_{s_1s_2}\cdot r_{s_3a_1}$ 1 at 4 p.e., 2 at 3·5 p.e., 12 at 2·5 p.e., remaining 45 < 2 p.e.

6. $F=r_{s_1a_1}\cdot r_{s_2a_2}-r_{s_1a_2}\cdot r_{s_2a_1}$ 1 at 3·5 p.e., 2 at 2·5 p.e., remaining 57 < 2 p.e.

The first kind of tetrad in this table is composed of two 'assembling' and two 'stripping' tests, and is designed to indicate whether these two classes of test depend on a single group-factor, or whether, on the contrary, there exists a factor in one class (or both) which does not function in the other. Since one coefficient in the left-hand product is the correlation between two 'stripping' tests, while the other is that between two 'assembling' tests, any super-correlation in either coefficient would tend to make the left-hand product greater than the right-hand and so produce a positive F. The actual distribution of the 120 tetrads, 'directed' in this way, indicates no such tendency. The F's are equally distributed on either side of approximately 0·6 times the probable error, i.e. in a way to be expected if the two kinds of test involve, as a class, no other than a single group-factor. Only three F's exceed 4 times the probable error, and of these, only one exceeds our standard of 4·5 times the probable error. All three are cases where $r_{s_1s_2}$ of the tetrad is the correlation between stripping 'wedges' and stripping 'containers' (0·48)—tests in which the movements associated with the operation of unscrewing are closely similar. This suggests the possibility of a small additional factor common to these two tests

—a suggestion, however, which is not confirmed when the 'stripping' tests are compared with one another (class 3 tetrads).

The second kind of tetrad is composed wholly of 'assembling' tests, i.e. of coefficients drawn from square A of Table XXII, and is designed to show whether there is evidence of a factor common to a certain pair (or pairs) of 'assembling' tests but absent in other pairs of 'assembling' tests. Of the fifteen tetrads, the largest is only 2·15 times the probable error, and the majority are under twice the probable error. The results thus indicate no evidence of factors within the 'assembling' group of tests other than the single group-factor to which their specific inter-correlation must be ascribed.

Similar evidence with respect to the 'stripping' tests is provided by our third type of tetrad. Again, there is no indication of any additional factor within this group, the largest F being under three times the probable error.

Tetrads in class 4 of our table are designed to indicate whether there may be a factor common to certain 'assembling' and 'stripping' tests which is not shared by other 'assembling' tests, i.e. tetrads in which two members are taken from square A and two from rectangle B of Table XXII. It follows mathematically, and as a logical deduction from our conclusions concerning the identity of the group-factor in 'assembling' and 'stripping', that, if the F's of class 1 tend to zero, so will those of class 4. At the same time, it seemed worth while to examine this class in order to see how far certain individual members of it deviate from zero—in particular, whether the *sameness* of the material (with consequent similarity of movement) in 'assembling' and 'stripping' introduces an additional factor. Again, no such factor comes to light, for of the 120 F's none attains to four times the probable error, and only two exceed three times the probable error; of the seventeen which exceed twice the probable error, eleven do so on account of the small negative correlations in rectangle B rather than to any positive correlation.

In class 5, the inter-correlations of 'assembling' tests which occur in class 4 are replaced by those of 'stripping' tests, i.e. two coefficients are taken from rectangle B and two from square C. Once more, they provide no evidence of additional group-factors, for none reaches our standard of $4\frac{1}{2}$ times the probable error. One, however, is approximately 4 times the probable error and is, therefore, suggestive. It is that tetrad which contains the correlation between stripping wedges and stripping containers—tests in which the possibility of a small additional factor has already been indicated.[1]

Finally, in class 6 we have tetrads in which the coefficients are drawn wholly from rectangle B of Table XXII ('assembling' *v.* 'stripping'). The largest F is below four times the probable error, and would be under twice, were it not for the small negative coefficient in the tetrad. With this class we complete the examination of every tetrad in the table. Nowhere has it produced definite evidence of other than a single group-factor peculiar to the routine tests as such.

(*b*) *Girls.* Table XXIII gives similar data for the girls' group. Application of the tetrad-difference criterion yields like results. Nowhere does the difference reach $4\frac{1}{2}$ times the probable error. Of four differences which are approximately four times the probable error, three owe their magnitude in part to the small negative correlations in the table rather than to any positive super-correlation. The remaining one is that in which the correlation of assembling screws with assembling wedges occurs, and it is *suggestive* of a further small factor common to these two tests. As against this view, however, the existence of such a factor is not evidenced in the boys' data. Neither does the additional factor common only to stripping wedges and stripping containers, which was suggested in the boys' data, find corroboration here.

3. CONCLUSION.

We must conclude that, after due allowance is made for the influence of 'general intelligence', the resulting specific correlations nowhere provide strong evidence of factors peculiar to the routine operations, as such, other than a single 'routine' factor upon which success at these operations, in so far as they exhibit specific correlation, must in part depend. Even where the operations consist in 'assembling' and in 'stripping' the same material, the specific correlation is no higher than can be reasonably attributed to the same factor as in the other routine tests.

The presence of small additional factors is at times suggested, but is nowhere definitely established in the present data. In our next section, however, there appears evidence of some specific correlation between certain 'mechanical' and 'routine' tests; but this, it will be seen, can in no wise be attributed to an additional 'routine' factor.

---

[1] In the tetrads of class 1.

C. RELATION OF THE 'ROUTINE' FACTOR TO THE 'MECHANICAL' FACTOR

1. THE QUESTION.

It remains to inquire how the 'mechanical' factor, disclosed in the mechanical assembling and mechanical aptitude tests, is related to the 'routine' factor of the routine assembling tests. Are these one and the same factor or are there two independent factors?

The answer is not immediately obvious. Both 'mechanical' assembling and 'routine' assembling involve the practical manipulation of material. Consequently, it is conceivable that this aspect of the work might introduce a 'motor' factor into both groups of assembling tests. On the other hand, the mechanical aptitude tests require no manual work, so that any factor common to these and to the assembling tests (either 'mechanical' or 'routine') could not be due to manual skill, as ordinarily understood. On this score, we should expect the factors to be different in the two cases. As against this view, however, there is the further consideration that skill in dealing mentally with the spatial elements out of which the problems of the 'mechanical' tests are built, and skill in manipulating the various pieces into position as required by the routine tests, may both depend on some underlying factor associated with the cognition of relations in space. These considerations, and the fact that the two groups show some correlation with one another (Tables XII and XIII), make it worth while to examine the relationship between the factors which have been found in each group.

2. FACTORS COMMON TO 'ROUTINE' AND 'MECHANICAL' TESTS.

Our examination of Tables XII and XIII, in Chapter v, has already indicated that, as a group, the routine 'assembling' tests correlate with the 'mechanical' tests to about the same extent as they correlate with the 'intelligence' tests, and that the 'stripping' tests correlate less, if anything, with the 'mechanical' tests than they do with the 'intelligence' tests (cf. rectangles Q and S with rectangle D of each table). A superficial examination of the tables suggests, therefore, that such correlation as is observed between these two groups may be wholly accounted for by the correlation which they exhibit in common with 'intelligence'. In other words, they do not suggest the presence of a wide group-factor common to 'mechanical' and 'routine' tests.

Application of the tetrad–difference criterion bears out the general indication, but is suggestive of group-factors in certain instances. Taking first the boys' data (Table XII), and comparing with one another tests of mechanical assembling, of routine stripping, and of 'intelligence'—i.e. tetrads formed by taking a coefficient from each of rectangles Q, A, D and E—of the twenty-four tetrad differences, none reaches our standard of 4·5 times the probable error, twenty-one are less than 3 times the probable error, eight are less than the probable error, and, although 'directed' so that a group-factor should produce a positive value, five are negative. Here, then, is no evidence of a factor peculiar to 'stripping' and 'mechanical' assembling, as such. One value, however, reaches 4·03 times the probable error and is, therefore, *suggestive* of a small factor common to the pair of tests concerned, viz. 'wiring' and 'stripping' wedges.

On comparing 'mechanical aptitude' with 'stripping', i.e. tetrads constituted of one coefficient from each of rectangles S, B, D and E, the F values again yield no positive evidence of group-factors, for none reaches 4·5 times, and fourteen of the available sixteen are under twice the probable error. One is 4·04 times the probable error. It is that in which, as before, the 'stripping' wedges test occurs and suggests the possibility of a factor, common to the test and to 'mechanical explanation' (test E).

Proceeding in similar fashion with the routine 'assembling' tests, and taking first tetrads of the kind formed of a coefficient from each of rectangles P, A, C, E, it is found that the values of the thirty F's distribute equally on either side of approximately 2·5 times the probable error, and all but one are positive. Four exceed 4 times—three of these exceed 4·5 times the probable error. Here, then, is more positive evidence of a group-factor (or factors) common to certain 'routine' and 'mechanical' assembling tests. The interesting point about this comparison is that the observed super-correlation does not occur between tests employing the same material for the two kinds of operation. Thus, the three F's which exceed 4·5 times the probable error are indicative of small factors common (i) to the 'mechanical' assembling of 'containers' and the 'routine' assembling of 'porcelains', and (ii) to the 'mechanical' assembling of 'porcelains' and routine 'wiring'.

The evidence of a group-factor appears most clearly in the tetrads which have yet to be examined, viz. those composed of one coefficient from each of rectangles R, B, C, E. Their distribution is given in Table XXV.

Table XXV.

Mid-value F/p.e.	+ 2·5	3·5	4·5	5·5	6·5
Frequency	4	4	9	1	2

The central value of the distribution (over 4 times the probable error) is seen to depart widely from zero and is thus indicative of a group-factor best located in rectangle R of the table (mechanical aptitude *v.* routine assembling).

An examination of corresponding data for the girls (Table XIII) may be summarized as follows:

(i) There is no indication of super-correlation in rectangles Q, S and R; for the relevant tetrad differences, although directed as before, are distributed equally on either side of zero between the limits of ± 4 times the probable error.

(ii) There is evidence of super-correlation in rectangle P; for the relevant 'directed' tetrads are all positive, their central value is approximately 2·3 times, three are approximately 4·5 times, two are 5·5 times, and two are 6·5 times the probable error. They thus indicate a group-factor (or factors) common to certain mechanical assembling and routine assembling tests.

The combined evidence of both tables indicates, therefore, the presence of a group-factor (or factors) common to the 'routine' assembling and the 'mechanical' tests—more marked in mechanical aptitude tests with the boys and in mechanical assembling tests with the girls. There is little evidence that such a factor extends into the 'stripping' tests.

3. THE 'ROUTINE' FACTOR DIFFERENTIATED FROM THE 'MECHANICAL' FACTOR.

(a) *In 'routine' assembling.* Had the tetrads which we have just examined indicated an entire absence of group-factors, the question with which this section opens, namely, whether the 'mechanical' factor is to be identified with the 'routine' factor, would now have been answered; for clearly, if members of one group of tests have nothing in common with members of the other, that which is common to members of the one cannot be the same as that which is common to members of the other. Since, however, our inquiry has disclosed that the mechanical tests and the routine tests may sometimes involve a common group-factor, further analysis becomes necessary before our question can be answered.

The matter may be put to a crucial test by examining tetrads of the kind $F = r_{m_1 m_2} \cdot r_{R_1 R_2} - r_{m_1 R_2} \cdot r_{R_1 m_2}$, where the m's are any two 'mechanical' tests, the R's are two 'routine' tests, and the r's are coefficients of 'specific' correlation.

Table XXVI.

'Specific' correlation between 'mechanical' and 'routine' tests, i.e. influence of the general factor removed from Table XII. Sixty boys. (Decimal points omitted.)

		Routine								
		Assembling					Stripping			
		S	We	P	C	Wi	S	We	P	C
Mechanical assembling	C	22	19	29 **P**	12	10	17	08 **Q**	16	12
	P	17	13	21	15	30	00	03	05	14
	Wi	03	01	23	11	16	−05	23	−04	12
Mechanical aptitude	E	33	25	36 **R**	22	45	07	27 **S**	16	08
	M	32	23	33	20	36	11	13	05	−08

AVERAGES.

P=0·16.   R=0·305.
Q=0·08.   S=0·10.

Table XXVII.

'Specific' correlation between 'mechanical' and 'routine' tests, i.e. influence of the general factor removed from Table XIII. Thirty-six girls. (Decimal points omitted.)

		Routine								
		Assembling					Stripping			
		S	We	P	C	Wi	S	We	P	C
Mechanical assembling	C	29	20	16	08	17	24	20	26	−23
	P	22	41	17 **P**	06	20	−27	24 **Q**	01	−16
	Wi	44	52	09	14	40	09	−06	14	−14
	T	28	38	31	15	59	−11	41	11	−08
Mechanical aptitude	E	25	12	−02 **R**	12	−02	−07	−07 **S**	04	−01
	M	15	30	15	08	28	−04	13	−06	−02

AVERAGES.

P =0·26.   R=0·14.
Q=0·04.   S = − 0·01.

The 'specific' correlation between the 'mechanical' and the 'routine' tests, required for this purpose, is given in Tables XXVI and XXVII. Incidentally, the specific correlation between the mechanical tests and the routine assembling tests, observed in these tables, and its relative absence from the 'stripping' tests, express in another way the results concerning group-factors arrived at in Section 2 above.

The specific inter-correlations of the mechanical tests and of the routine tests, which form the other members of the tetrad, have already been referred to and will be found in Tables XVI, XVII, XXII and XXIII.

The distribution of these tetrads from the boys' data, 'directed' as hitherto, where (i) both m's are mechanical aptitude tests, and (ii) both m's are mechanical assembling tests, are given in Table XXVIII.

Table XXVIII.

Mid-value F/p.e.	+ 0·5	1·5	2·5	3·5	4·5	5·5
Both m's 'aptitude' tests	2	4	4	4	2	4
Both m's 'mechanical' assembling	13	27	15	5	—	—

The presence of super-correlation is clearly shown in the first row of Table XXVIII. This means that the specific correlation between the mechanical aptitude tests *cannot* be attributed wholly to the same factor as that which produces the specific correlation between the routine assembling tests. In other words, the 'mechanical' factor cannot be identified with the 'routine' factor.

The super-correlation is less marked when the mechanical assembling tests are compared with the routine assembling tests, as shown in the second row of Table XXVIII. There is, however, a decided shift of the central value of F in the positive direction; and every one of the sixty F's is positive. Furthermore, many of the remaining tetrads of this general type, viz. those in which one m is a mechanical assembling test and the other is an aptitude test, provide distinct evidence of super-correlation. Thus, of 120 such tetrads from our boys' data, twenty-four exceed 3 times, and of these, four exceed 4 times and a further four exceed five times, the probable error; and there is a marked shift of the central value in the positive direction.

Similar results are observed in the data from the girls' group (Table XXVII). The distribution of the F's, where both m's are the aptitude tests, is given in Table XXIX.

As with the boys, the super-correlation is less marked when

mechanical assembling tests replace the aptitude tests. Of such tetrads only three exceed 3 times the probable error. At the same time, fifty-three of the available sixty are positive—the remaining seven being just below zero—so that, once again, the central value tends to a positive

Table XXIX.

	−	+				
Mid-value F/p.e.	0·5	0·5	1·5	2·5	3·5	4·5
Frequency	1	1	3	7	7	1

value rather than to zero.[1] To take, finally, those tetrads in which one m is a mechanical assembling test and the other is an aptitude test, nine of these exceed 3 times, while a further seven exceed 4 times the probable error. The conclusions to be drawn from the girls' results are thus in general agreement with those derived from the boys'.

(b) *In 'stripping'*. We have confined our examination, so far, to those routine tests in which the operation is that of 'assembling', because in these both the 'routine' factor and specific correlation with the mechanical tests were most in evidence. Since our examination of tetrads in the previous section of this chapter produced no evidence of important group-factors common to 'stripping' and the mechanical tests, it follows that where a group-factor is manifested in the former, it is not likely to be the same as that in the latter. The results obtained on examining the relevant tetrad differences, i.e. F's similar in type to those which we have just examined, but in which the R's are both 'stripping' tests, are in conformity with this view. The values of all *which exceed thrice their probable errors* have been calculated and are summarized from the boys' data in Table XXX.

Table XXX.

	+					
Mid-value F/p.e.	3·5	4·5	5·5	6·5	7·5	8·5
Both m's 'aptitude' tests	1	3	—	—	1	1
Both m's 'mechanical' assembling	10	3	3	1	—	—
One 'm' 'aptitude', the other 'assembling'	1	2	—	—	—	—
Total...	12	8	3	1	1	1

In many cases, the F values are seen to be too large to be assigned to 'chance'. This and the fact that those below 3 times the probable error are positive (and, consequently, so is their central value), point

---

[1] The 'tap' test has been omitted from this examination as having little in common with the other 'mechanical' tests. It was not taken by the boys.

to the conclusion that the specific correlation between the mechanical tests and such specific correlation as occurs between the 'stripping' tests are not due to the same factor.

To complete our comparison of 'routine' tests with 'mechanical' tests, there remain tetrads of the kind where one R is a 'routine' assembling test and the other is a 'stripping' test, the m's being mechanical tests as before. An examination of these leads to the same conclusion, for seventeen exceed 3 times, a further eight exceed 4 times, and a further four exceed 5 times the probable error; and there is the same general tendency of the remaining F's to distribute around a positive value rather than zero. As hitherto, the two factors are most clearly differentiated where the two 'mechanical' tests which enter into the tetrad are of the 'aptitude' type. Of the forty such F's, six exceed 3 times, a further six exceed 4 times, and a further three exceed 5 times the probable error, and all are positive.

A similar comparison of the data obtained from the girls leads to the same general conclusion; although owing to the larger probable error consequent on the smaller size of the group, the evidence by itself is of less statistical significance. It may be briefly summarized by saying that of all the tetrads in which either one or both R's are 'stripping' tests, thirty-three exceed 3 times, and of these five exceed 4 times, the probable error.

D. OBJECTIVE ANALYSIS OF 'ROUTINE' ASSEMBLING

In the light of our analysis we may now attempt to answer the question as to what are the abilities upon which success at routine assembling work depends, and in respect of which an individual must be measured, if we are to predict his capacity for this sort of work with any hope of success. It is clear that the term 'ability for routine assembling work' has no intelligible meaning unless the various operations which constitute 'assembling work' (or the assembling work in question) depend upon one and the same 'ability' in virtue of which an individual who does well at one of them will tend to do well at the others. Unless such a 'common core' exists, no measure of ability at one operation can afford the slightest indication of a person's ability at another. It is, therefore, of first importance for vocational guidance and selection, to determine whether such a 'common core' exists, and to secure an adequate measure of *this*. An exception would occur if ability at one operation were found to correlate perfectly with that at another (within the limits of experimental error). The 'common core' would then be co-extensive with the whole operation. Since perfect correlations are not found, the dependence of any given operation on the 'common core' can, at best, be only partial. For this reason, we have preferred the term 'factor' rather than 'ability' to denote such a 'core'. The mere sub-summing of a number of different operations under one term, such as 'assembling work', provides no reason for supposing that a 'common core' or 'group-factor' does in fact exist; nor for supposing the existence of only one such factor. Should there be more than one, the further question as to their relationship to each other arises. Do both, for example, run throughout the whole of the operations in question, or does one occur in one group (such as our 'routine' assembling operations) and the other in another (such as our 'stripping' operations)? Such questions, fundamental to any measurement of mental abilities, can be answered by experimental evidence alone. Where, however, subjective analysis is able to supplement this by offering a psychological explanation, there is a gain, not only in understanding, but also in generality: for the conclusion may then be extended to wherever the explanatory cause is seen to operate.

Of the common factors in routine assembling, only two emerge from the present analysis with any degree of certainty or generality. Of these, we have seen that one is of wider range than the other, and extends its influence beyond the assembling operations into the intelligence tests, and into the school examinations which depend largely on general intelligence. It is most reasonably identified with the same general factor as was observed to run throughout the tests of 'mechanical' assembling and of 'intelligence'.

The correlations with this general factor, shown in the last columns of Tables VII and IX, indicate that its influence is greater in the 'assembling' than in the 'stripping' operations, *each considered as a group* (cf. the average figures for the groups). But the coefficients for the individual tests show that it would be unsafe to apply this as a general rule. Neither do they suggest that 'saturation' with the general factor is dependent on the complexity of the operation, for the figures for the simple screwing operations (assembling and stripping 'screws') compare favourably with the others.

The other factor is restricted to the routine assembling operations. An indication of its magnitude and range is given in its correlations with these operations. These, determined from the specific correlations of Table XXII, are given in the last column of that table.[1] Its influence is seen to be greater in the 'assembling' than in the 'stripping' operations—a result confirmed by the data from the girls (cf. squares A and C of Table XXIII). In three of the four 'stripping' tests its influence is small. It follows that the measurement of this factor must be sought in the assembling rather than in the stripping type of test.

It is noteworthy that, although of greatly diminished influence in the stripping tests, it is not replaced by another factor. There is, for example, no evidence of a 'speed' factor running through the stripping tests (cf. the zero correlations in square D)—a result of obvious importance in the analysis of assembling work.[2]

On comparing the correlations of the 'routine' factor with those of the general factor (last columns of Tables VII and XXII), it is seen that the former enters into the assembling operations, as a group, to a much larger extent—the average being 0·53 and 0·23 respectively. Differences occur in the individual tests; but here, owing to the larger sampling error, we are on less secure ground.

In addition to this 'routine' factor, there has appeared some evidence for the existence of a third factor which, unlike the other, is not peculiarly associated with routine assembling as such, but which functions in both 'mechanical' and 'routine' assembling tests. Analysis suggests that this is not a new factor in our data, but the extension of one of the already determined factors into the other group. If, as seems reasonable, the routine factor be associated with the motor aspect of assembling work, the fact that in the boys (Table XXVI) 'routine assembling' correlates 'specifically' higher with 'mechanical aptitude' than with 'mechanical assembling' suggests the extension of the mechanical factor into the routine tests rather than the converse. This would be understandable, since both require the manipulation of objects in space—the one mentally, the other manually.

With the girls, the correlation is higher with the 'mechanical assembling' tests (Table XXVII, rectangle P). Seeing that these tests also involve the mechanical factor—and to a greater degree than with

---

[1] Owing to the small specific correlation with the 'mechanical' tests, and to the sampling error, such figures are only approximate.

[2] An important difference between 'assembling' and 'stripping' may be roughly expressed by saying that the former needed care, the latter speed.

the boys—such a result is not inconsistent with the above explanation. At the same time, it leaves open the possibility that the 'routine' factor may also have extended into the mechanical assembling tests—a not unlikely occurrence seeing that both involve manipulative work. But the specific correlations with the aptitude tests, referred to above, rule the routine factor out as a complete explanation, and it is not impossible that both factors may have played some part.

Finally, as was noticed in regard to the 'mechanical' tests, the intercorrelations of the 'routine' tests are far below unity. Indeed, to the lay mind the fact that the various routine operations are not more closely related than they turn out to be may seem the most surprising result of the whole investigation. Those familiar with the low correlations which have been generally observed between 'motor' tests will find, on the contrary, the present figures unexpectedly high—especially for the (routine) assembling operations. Seeing that the agreement between the tests is not perfect, we must suppose that in addition to the above-described factors, success at any given operation depends also partly on an element specific to the operation itself—or to the conditions under which it is performed. Such specific elements appear to play a larger part in the 'stripping' operations.

To sum up, success at routine assembling appears to depend on (i) general ability as measured by intelligence tests, (ii) a group-factor specially associated with the routine work, (iii) to a less extent, the 'mechanical' factor observed in mechanical assembling, and (iv) elements peculiar to each particular operation. Where the careful adjustment of parts tends to be replaced by mere speed of performance, as in 'stripping', the common factors tend to disappear, leaving the operation largely dependent on elements specific to itself. While further evidence is, of course, desirable, these conclusions appear to hold over a wide range of 'assembling ability' and of mental development—as witness the figures for 'total ability' over a period of practice, and for the backward group.

CHAPTER VIII

THE RELATION OF SIMPLE MANUAL TESTS
TO THE ROUTINE TESTS

A. AIM OF EXTENDING THE INQUIRY
INTO SIMPLER TESTS

The routine manual operations referred to in the preceding chapters are more complex in character than those which are generally adopted as laboratory tests of manual dexterity and which have often been employed in previous research on 'motor' ability.[1] The results examined so far suggest that the group-factor in the routine assembling and stripping tests may be associated with the complexity of the operation, and that, as the operation becomes less complicated, success depends less on the group-factor and more on the 'specific' factor peculiar to the test itself. They further indicate that where, as among the simpler stripping operations, the importance of the group-factor tends to diminish, its place is not taken by another group-factor, associated, for example, with 'speed' or 'simplicity'. At the same time, they hint at the possibility that where the operations are closely similar, as in unscrewing 'containers' and unscrewing 'wedges', the 'specific' factor may become the same in each, thereby causing some 'specific' correlation between the pair in question.

In view of these important indications, it is of obvious interest to determine how the routine operations investigated in the present research are related to the simpler types of manual activity referred to above. By thus extending our analysis, valuable light should be shed not only on the organization of these simpler, though nevertheless important, processes, but also on the nature of the group-factor in the more complex routine assembling and stripping tests. After the completion of the work described in the foregoing pages, such an extension of the inquiry was carried out and will be briefly described in the present chapter.

[1] As, for example, tapping at maximum speed, inserting pegs in holes, putting rings on a rod, turning a screw.

B. THE DATA COLLECTED

The following tests were given to fifty-nine elementary schoolboys similar in age and in educational attainment to those who provided the results examined in the previous chapters:[1]

1. ROUTINE ASSEMBLING TESTS.

As described in Chapter III, viz. the assembling of containers (C_a), of wedges (We_a) and of screws (S_a). In each case, the assembly of ten of the objects constituted one trial; in containers and wedges two trials, and in screws three trials, made the complete test.[2]

2. ROUTINE STRIPPING TESTS.

As in our previous investigations, stripping alternated with assembling in each of the above tests, thus yielding three stripping tests which will be referred to as C_s, We_s and S_s respectively.

3. SIMPLE MANUAL TESTS AS FOLLOWS.

(*a*) Threading beads (B), in which the subject was required to thread large beads on to a wire at maximum speed. The threading of twenty beads constituted one trial, three trials made the complete test.

(*b*) The turnbuckle test (T 1), in which the subject was required to screw up a turnbuckle (or wire-strainer) at maximum speed, involving twisting movements of finger and thumb combined with turning of the wrist.

(*c*) The turnbuckle test (T 2), in which the subject *un*screwed the turnbuckle as fast as possible.

(*d*) The rings test (R 1), in which the subject was required to place, as quickly as possible, curtain rings over a vertical wooden rod. The placing of twenty rings constituted one trial, and three trials made the complete test.

(*e*) The rings test (R 2), in which the rings were taken off the rod one at a time and replaced in a box at maximum speed; the 'taking off' alternating with the 'putting on' (in R 1), and the same number of trials constituted the complete test.

---

[1] The testing was done at a different school and by another person—Miss N. Samuel.

[2] The procedure was as described in Chapter III, with the exception that here the number of 'trials' was necessarily reduced.

4. General intelligence test (I).

All subjects were given the same test of general intelligence as was previously employed, viz. Spearman's "Measure of 'intelligence' for use in schools".

C. EXAMINATION OF RESULTS

1. Further evidence of the group-factor in routine assembling and stripping tests.

The inter-correlations of all the tests are given in Table XXXI. Once again, there is observed a positive correlation between the various tests which, in view of their negligible correlation with 'intelligence', cannot be wholly attributed to the general factor observable in intelligence tests. It remains to determine how far these correlations arise from a single group-factor or how far they indicate, on the contrary, the existence of more than one such factor.

Confining attention first to the assembling and stripping tests, i.e. to the coefficients in squares A, B and D, and calculating the tetrad difference of every possible tetrad in this part of the table, we observe that nowhere does this difference approach our standard of 4·5 times its probable error.[1] Here, then, is further evidence of the single group-factor running through the assembling and the stripping operations. Again, it is seen to play a larger part in 'assembling' than in 'stripping', as shown by the occurrence of the larger coefficients in square A.[2]

A similar result is found on combining the three assembling and the three stripping tests each into a single 'pool' or 'team'. The inter-correlations are as follows: three assembling tests *v.* another three assembling tests, 0·75; three stripping tests *v.* another three stripping tests, 0·43; three assembling tests *v.* three stripping tests, 0·48.[3] The ensuing tetrad difference is 0·0921 with a probable error of 0·05669.[4] Again, the difference is not statistically significant, and the inter-correlation of the 'pools' is best accounted for by a single group-factor.

2. Extension of the factor into simpler manual tests.

On turning to the inter-correlations of the simpler manual tests given in square F of Table XXXI, and examining individually all the

---

[1] By formula 15, Spearman's *The Abilities of Man*, p. xi.
[2] Cf. the data of Chapter vii.
[3] By Spearman's formula for the correlation of sums, *Brit. Journ. Psych.* v, 417.
[4] By formula 16, *op. cit.*

relevant tetrad differences in relation to their probable error, we find that in only two cases is the presence of super-correlation indicated.[1] They occur between the two turnbuckle tests (0·73) and between the two ring tests (0·50). In every other instance the inter-correlations of the simpler manual tests with one another, and with the assembling and the stripping tests, are adequately explained by the same group-factor as was found to run through the assembling and the stripping tests.

The same data may be summarized by first pooling (by averaging) the two pairs of tests which exhibit super-correlation, and then pooling into a single team, as before, members of the same group. The inter-correlations, with the two turnbuckle and the two ring tests 'pooled', are given in Table XXXII. The inter-correlations of the 'pooled' groups are as follows: three assembling *v.* three simple tests, 0·53; three stripping *v.* three simple tests, 0·56; three simple *v.* three simple tests, 0·57. Taking these in conjunction with the coefficients given in the last paragraph of (1) above, we obtain the following tetrad differences: (*a*) where two members of the tetrad are 'assembling' groups, and two are 'simple' groups, 0·1466 with probable error 0·05836, (*b*) where two members of the tetrad are 'stripping' groups and two are 'simple' groups, 0·0685 with probable error 0·03797.[2] In neither case does the difference signify other than a single factor common to all three classes of operation.

3. AN ADDITIONAL FACTOR IN CERTAIN 'SIMPLE' TESTS.

We have seen that if the correlation between the two turnbuckle tests (0·73) and between the two ring tests (0·50) be excluded, nowhere in Table XXXI does the tetrad difference exceed 4·5 times its probable error. Hence we have concluded that nowhere, except in these four tests, is there evidence of any factor other than a single group-factor. On examining the tetrad differences into which either the two turnbuckle tests, or the two ring tests enter,[3] fifteen are found to exceed 4·5 times their probable error.[4] Nine of these are tetrads composed of the two turnbuckle tests and two tests selected from the assembling and stripping groups, four are composed of the two ring

---

[1] I.e. correlation too high to be explained wholly by the same factor as that causing the other inter-correlations.

[2] By formula 16, *op. cit.*

[3] I.e. tetrads in which either the coefficient 0·73, or the coefficient 0·50, or both, enter.

[4] Of these, twelve exceed 6 times, and one exceeds 7 times, the probable error.

Table XXXI.

Inter-correlations of assembling, stripping and simple manual tests. Fifty-nine schoolboys. (Decimal points omitted.)

		Ca	Wea	Sa	Cs	Wes	Ss	B	T1	T2	R1	R2	I
Assembling	Ca	—	64 A	44	35	51 B	07	44	35	36 C	39	30	-03
	Wea	64	—	43	37	57	05	34	40	47	52	28	-01
	Sa	44	43	—	14	34	03	25	21	28	19	-10	-05
Stripping	Cs	35	37	14	—	33 D	10	21	35	27 E	20	14	01
	Wes	51	57	34	33	—	17	34	38	52	29	24	25
	Ss	07	05	03	10	17	—	32	28	22	16	21	22
Simple	B	44	34	25	21	34	32	—	36	32	29	36	19
	T1	35	40	21	35	38	28	36	—	73	44	24	-09
	T2	36	47	28	27	52	22	32	73 F	—	29	10	04
	R1	39	52	19	20	29	16	29	44	29	—	50	-05
	R2	30	28	-10	14	24	21	36	24	10	50	—	05

Table XXXII.

Inter-correlations of assembling, stripping and simple manual tests, with T tests and R tests 'pooled'. Fifty-nine schoolboys. (Decimal points omitted.)

		Ca	Wea	Sa	Cs	Wes	Ss	B	T	R
Assembling	Ca	—	64 A	44	35	51 B	07	44	36 C	35
	Wea	64	—	43	37	57	05	34	43	40
	Sa	44	43	—	14	34	03	25	25	05
Stripping	Cs	85	37	14	—	33 D	10	21	31 E	17
	Wes	51	57	34	33	—	17	34	45	27
	Ss	07	05	03	10	17	—	32	25	19
Simple	B	44	34	25	21	34	32	—	34	33
	T	36	43	25	31	45	25	34 F	—	27
	R	35	40	05	17	27	19	33	27	—

AVERAGES.

A = 0·50. D = 0·20.
B = 0·27. E = 0·28.
C = 0·32. F = 0·31.

tests and two selected from the assembling and stripping groups, and two are composed of the two turnbuckle tests and the two ring tests. Here the differences are too large in relation to their probable errors to be ascribed to a single group-factor. Neither can they be explained by a single additional factor common to the turnbuckle and ring tests, since the tetrads composed of these four tests themselves exhibit super-correlation. In the light of a subjective analysis of the tests considered in conjunction with the magnitude of the correlation coefficients, they are readily accounted for by two small additional factors, one common to the two turnbuckle tests, the other common to the two ring tests.[1] The close similarity of the movements involved would seem to account for the introduction of these additional factors.

D. SUMMARY

A group of manual tests comprising (*a*) routine assembling operations, (*b*) routine stripping operations, and (*c*) simple manual operations, together with a test of general intelligence, was given to fifty-nine elementary schoolboys.

The manual tests showed a general tendency to correlate positively with one another, but little, if any, correlation with general intelligence.

Examination of the correlation coefficients by the tetrad–difference criterion indicated:

(1) the existence of a group-factor common to the assembling and the stripping tests and playing a rather more important part in the former (the conclusions of Chapter VII are thus confirmed);

(2) the entry of the same group-factor into quite simple manual tests;

(3) where these simple tests involve very similar movements, an additional factor limited to such closely similar tests is introduced.

There are thus disclosed two kinds of group-factor in the various manual operations we have studied: (1) a single group-factor of wide generality running through all the operations, and (2) small additional factors of very restricted range common only to those simple manual tests which involve closely similar movements.

---

[1] Group-factors of such limited range are sometimes called 'specific' factors.

CHAPTER IX

THE MEASUREMENT OF ABILITY AT ASSEMBLING WORK

A. THE 'ABILITIES' IN ASSEMBLING WORK

How, we may now ask, do the analytical results bear on the practical task of estimating a person's suitability for assembling work? The success of this estimate will depend on (1) knowledge of the 'abilities' upon which success at the work depends, and (2) the accuracy with which these abilities are measured. Our analyses are clearly concerned with both.

Success at assembling work has been shown to depend on a complex of factors. Of these, one has been identified with that measured by tests of general intelligence. Thus far there is some justification for the practice, adopted by at least one large engineering firm, of selecting applicants for assembling work largely according to the standard reached on leaving school; for school attainment provides a rough and ready indication of general intelligence. But as the *sole* criterion of ability, it is seriously defective, since it entirely ignores those *special* abilities (or group-factors) which, we have shown, also determine success at this work. Particularly so as these prove to be the major factors in success. It follows that the mechanical and the routine tests will generally provide more valid criteria than will, by itself, any measure of general intelligence.

This means far more than the obvious fact that the best indication of ability at a given assembling operation is a test involving the operation itself. This the large specific element in each test renders true; but it hardly needs an elaborate analysis for its discovery. Usually, however, it is required to estimate ability for a general type of work rather than for any single operation. Moreover, even if the task of evaluating and standardizing tests of every operation within a given field of assembling work were possible, it would be of little service in vocational guidance, for the *particular* demands which the future will make on a person in any given sphere of work must remain unknown. It is here that the analysis has its most direct bearing, since it indicates the mental elements, or factors, according to which the various kinds of assembling work may be most usefully analysed and classified, and in respect of which individuals must be measured if the resulting scores are to possess general validity within the class of operations to which they apply. These, as we have already seen, consist of the general factor referred to above together with two group-factors. Further research may, of course, disclose other factors in operations which fall outside the range of our present tests.

Briefly, the present results, coupled with our previous study of mechanical aptitude,[1] mean that the various engineering occupations (including, under this heading, the work of the assembling room) may be broadly and appropriately classified according to the demand which they make on the individual's general intelligence (or more correctly the general factor), his mechanical aptitude (or more correctly the mechanical factor) and his routine assembling ability (or more correctly the routine factor). The higher branches of engineering will demand the first two, but little, if any, of the third; the lower branches, consisting of straightforward assembling work, will require more especially the third; the intermediate branches, including repair work and more difficult assembling work, will require in varying proportions all three. These will be further divisible according to the extent to which success is conditioned by each of the factors—its 'saturation'. Where the work involves the mere repetition of a group of simple movements, in which the careful adjustment of parts to one another by touch is not called for, it will probably fall outside any of these classes, since neither factor appears to enter to any appreciable extent into these simpler operations. Here, owing to the large 'specific' element, a 'sample' test of the operation itself would seem to provide the best indication of ability. Fortunately, it is in this kind of work that such tests find most convenient application.

Experiment alone can substantiate and fill in the details of this broad classification. It serves, here, to illustrate the lines along which classification may most successfully proceed in the light of our results and, as such, provides a useful starting point. Above all, it supplies the elements according to which alone (within the scope of the inquiry) coefficients of 'validity' can be rightly interpreted.[2] It thus indicates

---

[1] Published in the writer's *Mechanical Aptitude* (London: Methuen and Co.).

[2] The 'validity' of a test is determined by its correlation with some known criterion of ability at the work. Much misunderstanding of experimental results in this field arises from the fact that the ability measured by the test and that measured by the criterion do not function in unitary fashion and so cannot be compared in the direct way so often attempted.

the path along which the experimental counterpart of the present work, viz. the determination of valid tests of vocational ability, may fruitfully proceed.

B. PRACTICAL REQUIREMENTS FOR MEASUREMENT

Besides indicating the factors to be measured, the foregoing analysis has an important bearing on the problem of measuring them; for it has indicated the magnitude of the correlation between each test and the group-factor which it is required to measure. These show how far the various tests are likely to provide an accurate measure of this factor.

It is seen that on the whole the mechanical tests exhibit higher correlation with the mechanical factor than do the routine tests with the routine factor; consequently, in their present form, a greater accuracy of measurement (of the factor in question) may be expected from the former tests than from the latter. But nowhere are these correlations sufficiently high to permit of accurate measurement from a single test.[1]

The remedy must be sought either in improving the test by raising its correlation with the factor, or by using a team of tests. In either case the needed condition is high correlation with the factor to be measured and low correlation with any other factor. Here, again, the 'mechanical' tests are seen to be better off than the 'routine' tests, for in the former the correlation with the group-factor shows a greater superiority over that with the general factor.[2]

The direction along which test improvement and team construction should proceed is also indicated in the results of the object analysis. The latter shows that where it is required to measure the mechanical factor, the above conditions are best fulfilled in the 'aptitude' type of test and in the more difficult of the assembling type; where the measurement of the routine factor is required, they are best fulfilled in the routine assembling tests, and especially in the 'wedges' and 'wiring' tests. These, then, will be the kind out of which to build suitable teams.

A reduction in the size of the team, and, consequently, in the time

---

[1] The accuracy with which a 'factor' can be measured is not to be confused with the accuracy with which a test will measure the whole operation which it is designed to measure. The former is indicated by the correlation with the factor, the latter by the correlation with itself—the 'reliability' coefficient.

[2] The remarks in this and the preceding paragraph apply more especially to the *aptitude* type of mechanical test. In the case of mechanical assembling, and routine assembling, the saturations with their respective factors are about equal.

required to administer it, will be made possible by increasing the 'saturation' of the constituent tests with the group-factor which it is required to measure. Here the objective results—of prime importance—may well be supplemented by subjective analysis. Improvement in the required direction may then be sought by so modifying the old tests, or devising new, that they include, so far as possible, only those processes which depend on the group-factor.

C. NORMS AND GROUP DIFFERENCES

1. NORMS OF PERFORMANCE.

A complementary step to the securing of accurate measures is the accurate comparison of one person's ability with another's. For this purpose knowledge of the average performance of the group to which the person belongs is convenient. While our groups were too small to yield highly reliable norms of this kind, they supply a rough and ready means of comparison for those who may wish to secure further results with the tests. The average scores made by our various groups, together with the standard deviations, are, therefore, given in Table XXXIII. The grouping is according to school attainment. This, however, is seen to agree throughout with the scores at the general intelligence test. Those subjects who were unable to take every test were necessarily excluded from our correlational data. Hence, the total number of subjects in the latter sometimes falls below that in Table XXXIII.

2. GROUP DIFFERENCES.

(a) *Sex*. No strict comparison between the sexes as regards ability at the assembling tests is possible, since nowhere have we two groups of the same average age and general intelligence. The two groups which most nearly satisfy the condition as regards intelligence are class II boys (av. score 112·7) and class IIB girls (av. score 111·5). In these the boys are superior in three of the five 'mechanical' tests and in six of the nine routine assembling tests. Seeing that the boys' average age is 1 year 1 month less than the girls', these figures suggest a general superiority of the boys over the girls in the 'mechanical' and 'routine' factor at this age. Some advantage in the tests would, of course, result from the slight superiority in 'intelligence' shown by these particular boys; but this is probably more than offset by their much younger age.

Table XXXIII.

Average scores and standard deviations for different school groups.

(9/6 = 9 min. 6 sec., otherwise seconds.)

| | 'Mechanical' | | | | | | 'Routine' | | | | | | | | | G.I.* | Age (yrs. mos.) |
| | Assembling | | | | Aptitude | | Assembling | | | | | Stripping | | | | | |
	C	P	Wi	T	E	M	50 S	50 We	10 P	50 C	5 Wi	50 S	50 We	10 P	50 C		
Boys																	
Class I																	
No. of subjects	35	35	28	—	35	35	36	36	36	35	35	36	36	34	35	33	36
Average	9/6	22/24	9/57·6	—	7·54	12·43	3/37	12/27·5	14/46	12/19·8	9/27	1/28·9	3/26·7	2/36	4/55·6	128·2	13/2·7
St. deviation	8/30·6	10/59·4	3/27	—	3·05	4·21	33·7	2/29·4	4/9	1/46	2/1	15·4	27·0	26·7	37·9	12·5	8·68
Class II																	
No. of subjects	34	36	31	—	35	35	37	37	37	36	35	37	37	33	36	35	37
Average	12/46	28/16	9/53·4	—	6·49	18·3	3/43	13/44	15/42	14/9·5	11/13	1/48·1	3/50·5	3/10	5/27·3	112·7	11/9·3
St. deviation	10/3	10/54·6	3/15·6	—	3·16	6·47	37·4	2/10	6/58	3/39	2/38·4	18·1	41·6	51	40·4	14·3	6·18
Girls																	
Class I																	
No. of subjects	—	—	—	—	—	—	13	13	—	—	—	13	13	—	—	13	13
Average	—	—	—	—	—	—	3/30·7	12/29·4	—	—	—	1/19·3	3/13·5	—	—	122·9	19/9
St. deviation	—	—	—	—	—	—	44·7	2/8·4	—	—	—	16·6	30·7	—	—	8·26	3·61
Class I A																	
No. of subjects	—	—	—	—	—	—	26	26	—	—	—	26	26	—	—	26	26
Average	—	—	—	—	—	—	3/54·3	13/29·2	—	—	—	1/44·6	3/45·3	—	—	114·2	12/11·3
St. deviation	—	—	—	—	—	—	39·5	2/47·4	—	—	—	18·2	28·6	—	—	10·7	9·3
Class II A																	
No. of subjects	17	16	16	21	21	21	21	21	21	21	21	21	21	21	21	21	21
Average	19/34	40/57	8/50	2/27	7·38	7·4	3/59·1	13/9·6	19/15	16/21	11/37	1/44·9	3/50·8	3/16	5/30·1	115·6	12/10·7
St. deviation	9/28·6	12/21·2	3/36·1	1/40·7	2·38	3·07	37·62	2/5·5	7/11·8	2/49·5	2/57·5	18·86	28·62	59·6	49·99	11·22	5·81
Class II B																	
No. of subjects	13	10	7	15	15	15	20	20	15	15	15	20	20	15	15	20	20
Average	19/54	46/11	9/24	2/25	6·6	7·13	4/15·9	13/37	17/12	16/41	11/12	1/49·9	3/46·8	3/19	5/29	111·5	12/10·3
St. deviation	12/43·8	4/41	3/24·1	1/34·1	1·93	2·96	35·5	1/55·8	5/24	3/23·7	2/24·8	19·9	19·5	41·4	47·5	10·25	8·0
Backward class																	
No. of subjects	12	5	14	9	8	8	22	22	8	8	18	22	22	8	8	22	22
Average	19/12	44/46	9/0·5	2/51·6	5·38	5·63	4/57·6	17/36·4	13/25·5	16/24	17/35·5	1/49·1	3/56·3	2/50·25	6/25·3	98·7	19/4
St. deviation	14/12·6	8/9·4	3/54·3	1/40·2	1·41	5·38	1/53·8	4/33·6	54·8	2/33·2	10/30·3	27·65	34·67	25·16	23·73	13·3	8·2

* G.I. = General Intelligence. See C. Spearman, *A Measure of 'Intelligence' for Schools* (London: Methuen and Co.).

This is confirmed when we compare the same group of boys with class II A girls, where the superiority as regards 'intelligence' is now with the girls. Here, again, the boys are superior in three of the five 'mechanical' tests and in eight of the nine 'routine' tests, although 1 year 1·4 months younger, and of lower average intelligence.

Comparison with the older, class I, group of boys is less satisfactory on account of greater differences in age and in 'intelligence'. They are superior throughout to the oldest group of girls who took all the tests (class II A), but they are also decidedly superior in the intelligence test (123·2 against 115·6) and in age (by four months). Both of these factors would tend to bring about some superiority in the assembling tests.

Only four 'routine' tests could be taken by the older girls of classes I and I A. Of these, class I closely approximates to class I boys in 'intelligence' (122·9 *v.* 123·2), but is 6·3 months older in age. It is superior in three of the four tests. Yet this may be due to the superiority in age. Class I A is inferior to class I boys in all four tests—but it is also inferior in age and in 'intelligence'.

Thus, although the research was not specially planned to indicate sex differences, and the groups are too small for definite general conclusions, the figures suggest in the younger groups a superiority of the boys over the girls in those factors especially associated with 'mechanical' and 'routine' assembling. In the older groups the difference appears to be less—if it exists at all; but there the issue is complicated by age differences and the restricted nature of the data.

(*b*) *Development.* A comparison between 'normal' groups of different ages indicates a general increase in ability at both 'mechanical' and 'routine' tests with age. Of the boys, the older group is superior to the younger in all except the 'mechanical' wiring, and the 'mechanical' models tests. Among the girls, the oldest group is superior to all the others in all the four tests taken. The next oldest (class I A) is superior to the younger groups in three.

The remaining 'normal' girls (II A and II B) were divided on a difference of school attainment and intelligence rather than of age—the difference in the latter being only 0·4 month. The scores are higher for the upper group in five of the six 'mechanical' tests and in five of the nine 'routine' tests.

Part of this increase in ability with age must, of course, be attributed to the increase in 'intelligence' which is also observed. The figures throw no light on how far development in the operations tested may be due to general mental development and how far to growth in the special factors involved. That they should increase together from one age group to another is in agreement with their observed correlation within the (fairly homogeneous) 'age' groups of our correlation tables.

The most interesting comparison is with the 'backward' girls—as judged by school attainment and the 'intelligence' test. Unfortunately the number able to take some of the tests is very small and there is no 'normal' group of exactly the same average age. It is noteworthy, however, that they do better than class II B in three of the 'mechanical assembling' tests, and in three of the 'routine' tests. It is clear, therefore, that they are far less retarded in these assembling operations than in 'intelligence' and in their work at school, for in these they fall far behind the standard of class II B. This affords grounds for believing that, although incapable at school work requiring a fair degree of general intelligence, they may prove satisfactory in work demanding 'special' abilities such as those which enter into the assembling operations.

PART III

DYNAMIC FUNCTIONS

CHAPTER X

ABILITY AND PRACTICE IN 'ROUTINE' OPERATIONS

A. PRACTICE CURVES OF ADULTS

1. INDIVIDUAL CURVES.

Some of the more interesting individual curves of our adult subjects, showing the time scores made in each of their eleven practices at the routine operations, are given in figs. 2–9.[1] For ease of comparison all the individual curves are placed within the same axes in figs. 10 and 11.[2] The practice period was planned to begin on a Monday and to continue daily, with the omission of Saturdays and Sundays, until (and including) the following Monday week. All subjects completed the eleven practices; but all were not able to conform exactly to this plan as regards dates. A break in the daily practice is indicated in the graphs of figs. 2–9 by a broken line.

It will be remembered that a practice consisted in alternately assembling and stripping a given number of objects for a given number of times. The graphs, throughout, show the average time required to effect the assembling (or stripping) of the given number of objects once. Thus the ordinates of figs. 2 and 10 are the average times required to assemble ten screws on each of the successive days of practice; i.e. one-tenth of the total time actually spent in practice, since this consisted in assembling, on each occasion, 100 screws (in groups of ten). Similarly, the graphs for 'porcelains' show the average time

[1] It has been found impossible to present all the curves that will be referred to in this chapter. See footnote to p. 49.
[2] The curves of figs. 10 and 11 have been smoothed by averaging each three consecutive days: thus the first point is the average of days 1, 2 and 3, the second point is the average of days 2, 3 and 4, and so on.

to assemble (or strip) five of these objects (a convenient unit of work for this material), whereas the total number assembled at a single practice was twenty (in groups of five). Similar remarks apply to the curves of practice at the other operations. They should be borne in mind when comparing the curves for one operation with those for another. It should also be noted that the unit of ability, and of practice, used throughout, is the time required to do a given quantity of work—not the work done in a given time.

(*a*) '*Screws.*' Before examining the general features of these curves—best shown by superimposing them into a single composite curve—it is worth looking at their more important individual characteristics, confining attention, first, to those subjects who practised the assembling and stripping of screws—figs. 2, 3 and 10. Of these, the curves of W are interesting as being those of the slowest subject in this group, both in the initial and the final practices, and in 'total ability' as measured by his total (or average) performance over the whole eleven practices.

Notwithstanding his poor ability in both 'assembling' and 'stripping', this subject makes the greatest absolute improvement in both operations. An interesting feature of both his curves is their step-like course in the early stages. Thus, in the 'assembling' operation, there is a marked improvement on the second day but none on the third. Slight improvement appears on the fourth, followed by a rapid and large improvement on the fifth with no improvement on the sixth; after this improvement takes a more steady course, and the slow regular descent of the curve closely approximates to that seen in the curves of some of the quicker subjects (cf. the latter stages of Mu).

In contrast with this step-like and somewhat erratic course is the extremely gradual and almost straight-line descent of the curves of our fastest subject, Mu. This curve also differs from the former (and most others) in suggesting that the limit of improvement was reached fairly early in the practice period. In neither operation is there any improvement after the sixth day (i.e. day 8 on the graph).

Differing again from either of these is the assembling curve of M. If we omit the fall-off on the sixth day (which may have been due to the week-end rest), the shape of this curve resembles more closely than any other (for this operation) that of the 'ideal' (or 'typical') curve of practice, viz. one in which the rate of improvement is maximal at first and constantly decreases until the limits of practice are reached

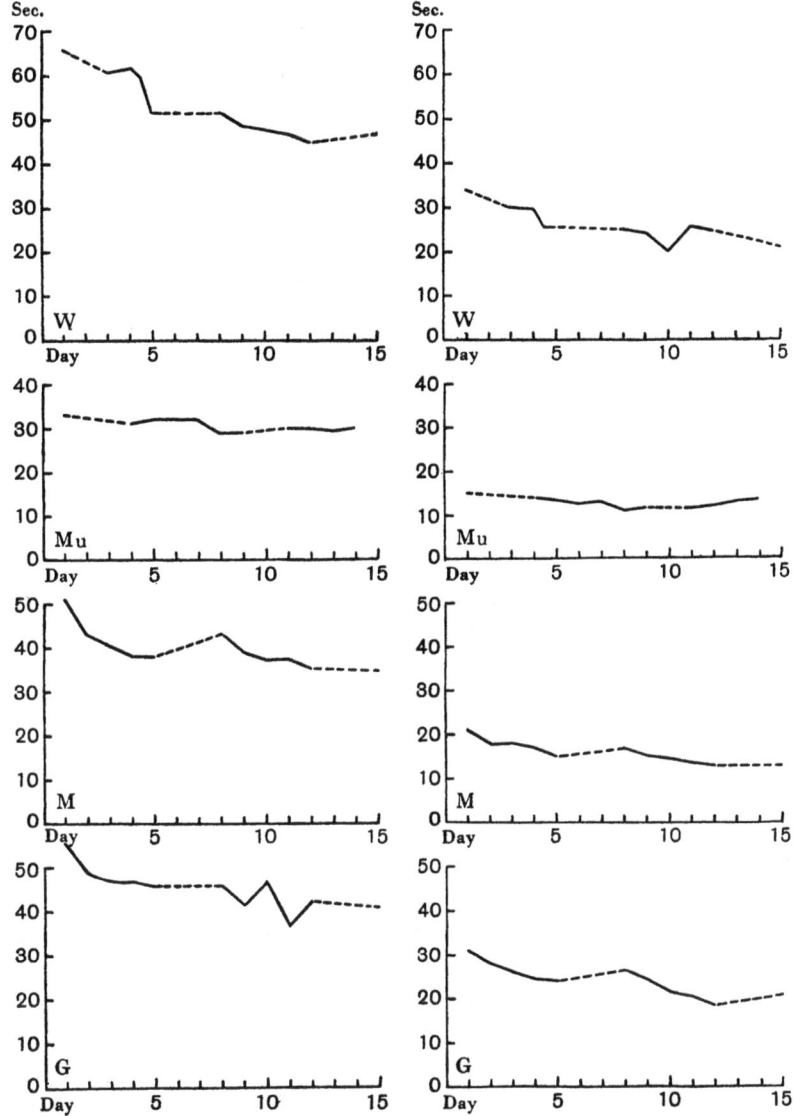

Fig. 2. Individual practice curves.
Average time to assemble ten screws.

Fig. 3. Individual practice curves.
Average time to strip ten screws.

and the curve assumes a horizontal direction. The first half of G's 'assembling' curve also approximates to this ideal type. The second part is rather jagged, but would, if smoothed out, represent very fairly a continuance of the first.

The assembling curves of H, M and I all show a marked fall-off in ability in the first day following the two days' rest which occurred in the middle of the practice period. In each case, the two parts into which the curve is thus sharply divided—associated with 'learning' and 're-learning' respectively—closely resemble one another. A similar loss in ability is sometimes observed after the second rest period. This may be partly due to the well-known 'Monday' effect. It is not characteristic of all subjects; neither, where observed, does it always appear consistently after both periods of rest.

(b) '*Porcelains.*' To turn from the simplest to the most complex of the operations, that of assembling porcelains—noteworthy features of these curves (figs. 4, 5 and 11) are, (1) the very irregular (though clearly marked) course which improvement takes with the weaker as compared with the quicker subjects,[1] and (2) the short steep initial fall which is seen in the curves of the latter. Our slowest subject, K, was remarkably clumsy, took over 33 min. to assemble the first five porcelains (as against the average time of 6 min. 7 sec.), damaged his fingers with the screwdriver, and showed marked emotion. In both 'assembling' and 'stripping', maximum improvement occurs on the second day of practice, followed by further marked improvements in 'assembling' on the fourth (after two days' rest). After the fourth day, progress is slow and shows much irregularity in the later practices at the 'assembling' operation. Initially ranking thirteenth (and lowest) in both operations, he finished eleventh at 'assembling' and third at 'stripping'. While his performance at 'assembling' is clearly slow throughout, his initially bad start in both operations seems to have been partly due to strongly toned feeling, accompanying the expressed belief that he 'was no good with his hands'.

In our next two 'slowest' subjects, S (whose total performance ranked twelfth in 'assembling', eleventh in 'stripping') and Wa (whose ranks were eleven and thirteen respectively), the irregularities are more evenly distributed throughout the curve, and the latter would more nearly approximate to a straight line if smoothed out.

The assembling curves of our more normal subjects tend to fall into

[1] Fig. 11 has been smoothed, see footnote 2, p. 107.

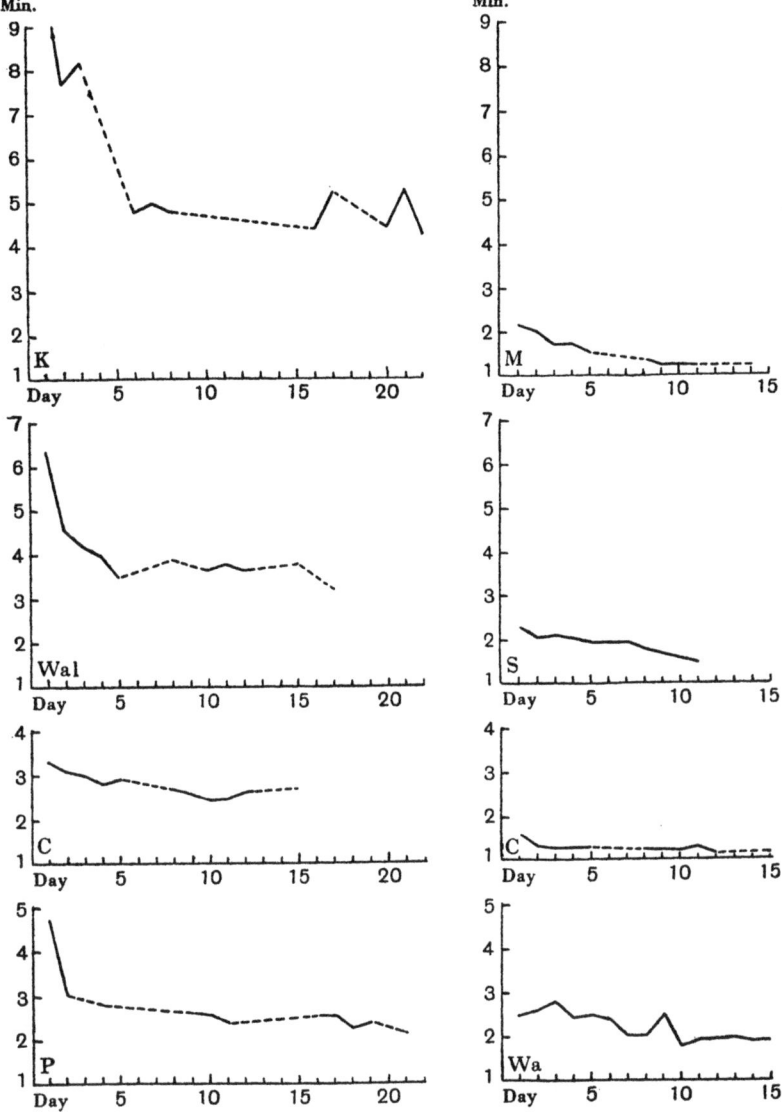

Fig. 4. Individual practice curves.
Average time to assemble five porcelains.

Fig. 5. Individual practice curves.
Average time to strip five porcelains.

two clearly marked phases, viz. a short period of steep descent followed by a longer period of much more gradual slope. Both parts approximate to a straight line and the change in direction is abrupt. The point of division occurs sometimes at the second day of practice, as in the curve of Wal (fig. 4), sometimes at the third day, and sometimes at the fourth day. Of the three abnormally slow subjects referred to above, it is clearly seen at the fourth practice with K. In the curves of S and Wa, the irregularities tend to mask the general direction, although similar points of division are suggested at the sixth day of practice in S and the fifth in Wa. Where the initial period lasts longer, it is less steep and the transition is less abrupt.

An interesting departure is seen in the curve of C (fig. 4), where the initial phase is absent. C is the present writer. As such he had watched the work of others and had devoted some attention to the analysis of movements (including the causes of success and failure) before beginning practice. Consequently, the work was approached with a clearer idea of the order, pattern and nature of the movements required. This suggests that during the initial steep phase learning is chiefly concerned with the cognitive aspect of the operation, while the succeeding phase of gradual descent marks the progress of its more purely motor side. In other words, in the first period the subject is mainly occupied in learning *about* the requisite movements, while in the second he is developing skill in their accurate and rapid performance.[1] The initial phase is particularly marked in the curves of Wal and P, both of whom gave careful attention at first to the method of handling the material, i.e. to one of the matters concerned on the 'cognitive' side.

P (fig. 4) is the fastest subject at this operation. He started fourth, rose to first place at the second practice, and maintained this position afterwards. He also made the greatest percentage improvement (i.e. gain in speed expressed as a percentage of his initial score), and ranked fifth in 'absolute' improvement. The short steep initial phase and subsequent smooth descent in his curve contrast strongly with the curves of the slower subjects. His 'stripping' curve is also seen to be one of the smoothest.

M showed the greatest 'absolute' improvement (omitting the very abnormal performance of K) and made the second highest percentage improvement. His curve more nearly resembles in shape the 'ideal' curve of practice than does any other in this group. In 'stripping' he

---

[1] For a fuller description see Chapter xv, where the 'cognitive' aspect is shown to consist very largely in acquiring knowledge of the 'characters' of the movements.

showed similar capacity for improvement, ranking second on the absolute scale, third on the percentage scale (fig. 5). The horizontal direction taken by his 'stripping' curve towards the end suggests that the limits of improvement had been attained. It contrasts, in this respect, with the 'stripping' curve of S which is seen to fall steadily in an almost straight line right up to the last day of practice (fig. 5).

The stripping curves of C and Wa (fig. 5) are interesting as being those of subjects who showed least improvability (both 'percentage' and 'absolute'). They differ strikingly in smoothness. C, it will be remembered, was the present writer, who had the opportunity to reflect on the operation and to handle the material in a casual fashion (for analytical purposes), before beginning this period of regular practice under test conditions. His curve suggests the tail-end of a practice period which had begun (*mentally*) before the first day of the practice proper. Wa's, on the other hand, represents from the beginning the efforts of a subject who was inherently weak at the operation (he also ranked lowest on 'total' ability).

(c) '*Containers*.' Some of the more interesting individual curves of practice at assembling 'containers' are given in fig. 6. The fastest subject for the whole period (total ability) was Wi. She started third and rose to first place on the third day of practice. Some fall-off is seen on the next two days, followed by marked improvement on the Monday after the week-end rest, when she regains the first place. This she maintained on the Tuesday, Thursday and Friday which followed, but dropped to second place on the Wednesday—a day which appears on the graph as the centre of a 'plateau'. After this the curve falls sharply to its lowest point. On the last day of practice, she did less well and dropped to third place. The curve consists, broadly, of three fairly rapid slopes separated by two plateaux—a course which we formerly described as 'step-like'.

L was the second fastest subject as measured on the total practice.[1] As compared with Wi, his progress is more rapid at first, is less evenly spread over the whole period, and appears to reach its limit more rapidly. The sharp initial fall in the curve (seen also in Ro, and Fl) suggests a distinction between the 'cognitive' and 'motor' aspects of the operation similar to that noticed above in the 'porcelain' curves. Unlike Wi, L shows a decided fall-off after the first rest period. Apart from this, the general course of improvement is more regular.

[1] It has been impossible to show all the curves here. See footnote to p. 49.

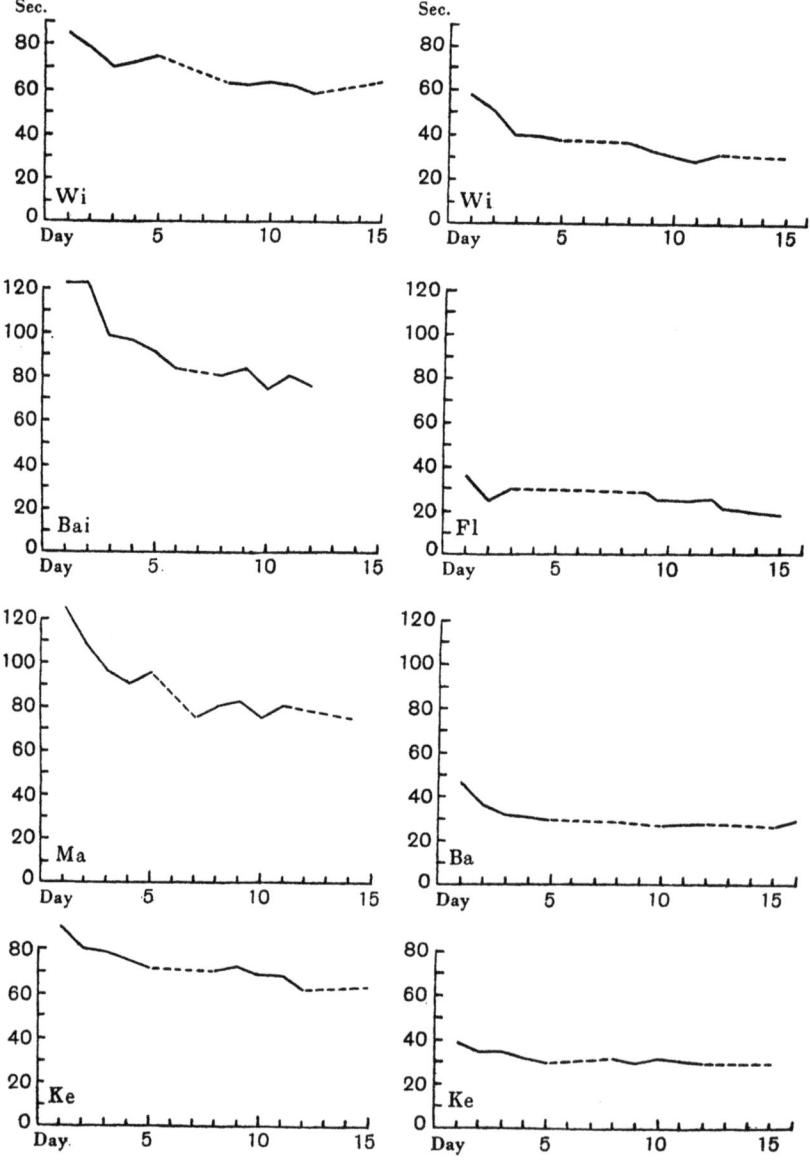

Fig. 6. Individual practice curves. Average time to assemble five containers.

Fig. 7. Individual practice curves. Average time to strip five containers.

Bai (fig. 6) was the slowest at this operation. She started eighth, fell to ninth on the second day of practice, and remained low (usually ninth) for the remainder of the period. Nevertheless, her curve indicates much improvement—a very sharp fall after the second day followed by a much more gradual, though regular, improvement up to the seventh day. The curve becomes more irregular as the limits of improvement were approached. The general shape suggests that the best score—made on the tenth day of practice—marked the beginning of a plateau rather than the actual limit. The slow irregular progress made at first as compared with the steep initial slope seen in the curves of faster subjects, and its more gradual shading off into the later stages (seen also in the curve of our next slowest subject, Ma), are remindful of similar differences which were observed in the 'porcelain' assembling curves.

The curve of Ma ('initially' ninth, 'terminally' eighth, 'total' ability eighth) is remarkable for its smooth rapid descent, approximating to the ideal type, during the first week, and the great gain shown on the Monday following the first rest period (fig. 6). After this no further progress is made until the last day, and the jagged character which the curve now assumes contrasts strongly with its smooth beginning—a contrast observable in several other cases.

Ma and Dr show the greatest 'improvability', ranking respectively first and second on 'absolute' improvement, and conversely on 'percentage' improvement. When smoothed out, their curves both resemble more closely than any other the typical curve.

Ba and Ke (fig. 6) have the two smoothest curves. In both, progress is more rapid at first, with some irregularity towards the end. Ba's best score was made on the seventh day. Up to this point the curve is remarkably smooth. The introspections suggest that some loss of interest occurred later on, owing partly to failure to improve on this score. This may have been a factor in causing the sudden rise in the curve which occurs on the ninth day. The indications that the limits of improvement had been reached are far less definite in the curve of Ke.

In contrast with the steady course of improvement shown in these cases, is the very irregular curve of Ro. Despite its apparently irregular course, definite progress is made and appears at regular intervals, namely initially and after each period of rest. Two explanations are possible. This subject ranked highest 'initially' and, in agreement with the general rule that those who do best at first (in these operations) show least improvement, she made little progress, as compared with the others. Consequently, her curve as a whole may be taken to represent merely the tail-end of the practice curve which, as we have already seen, tends to become jagged as it approaches the limits of improvement. Against this view is the large improvement shown on the last day and its regular appearance after each period of rest. This, together with the general behaviour of the subject, suggests the alternative (or additional) explanation, that initially and after each rest came a fresh burst of interest which resulted in some progress for the time being but which tended to wane as the days went on.

On turning to the 'stripping' curves (fig. 7), many features similar to those which appear in the assembling curves are to be seen. The same relatively steep initial fall followed by a much more gradual decline reappears in many of the curves—as shown in those of Fl and Wi in fig. 7.

A general similarity of shape between the 'assembling' and the 'stripping' curves of the same subject is often observable, and the general tendency for the 'stripping' curves to be smoother than those of 'assembling' is again evident.[1] Those of Ba and Ke (fig. 7) are again exceptionally smooth. The initial retardation of progress is again apparent in Bai. The curve of Dr also approaches more nearly to the 'ideal' shape.

Fl (fig. 7) was the fastest subject as measured on 'total' ability. He likewise ranked first 'initially' and 'terminally', and maintained this position almost throughout. For one starting so high, he showed a fair amount of improvement, ranking fifth 'absolutely' and third by the 'percentage' method. The rapid progress at first followed by the long plateau extending to the seventh practice is noteworthy. A similar, though shorter, plateau is seen in the course of our second fastest subject, Ma; but here the initial period of descent lasts much longer. Similar plateaux between periods of fairly rapid progress are found in the curves of Ro and L.

Wi (fig. 7) showed the greatest 'absolute' improvability. Most of the progress (roughly two-thirds) was made in the first three days.

[1] In comparing the two operations it must be remembered that 'stripping' is a much shorter operation than 'assembling'; to get a rough comparison on a common time basis the ordinates (and consequently the gradients) of the 'stripping' curves must be approximately doubled. Even so, the operations still differ in the total time spent at practice, as do the individuals, the common unit of practice being the number of objects assembled.

This part of the curve closely resembles in slope and shape what we have called the 'initial' phase. This phase is absent from the curve of Ke (fig. 7)—the subject showing least 'improvability'.

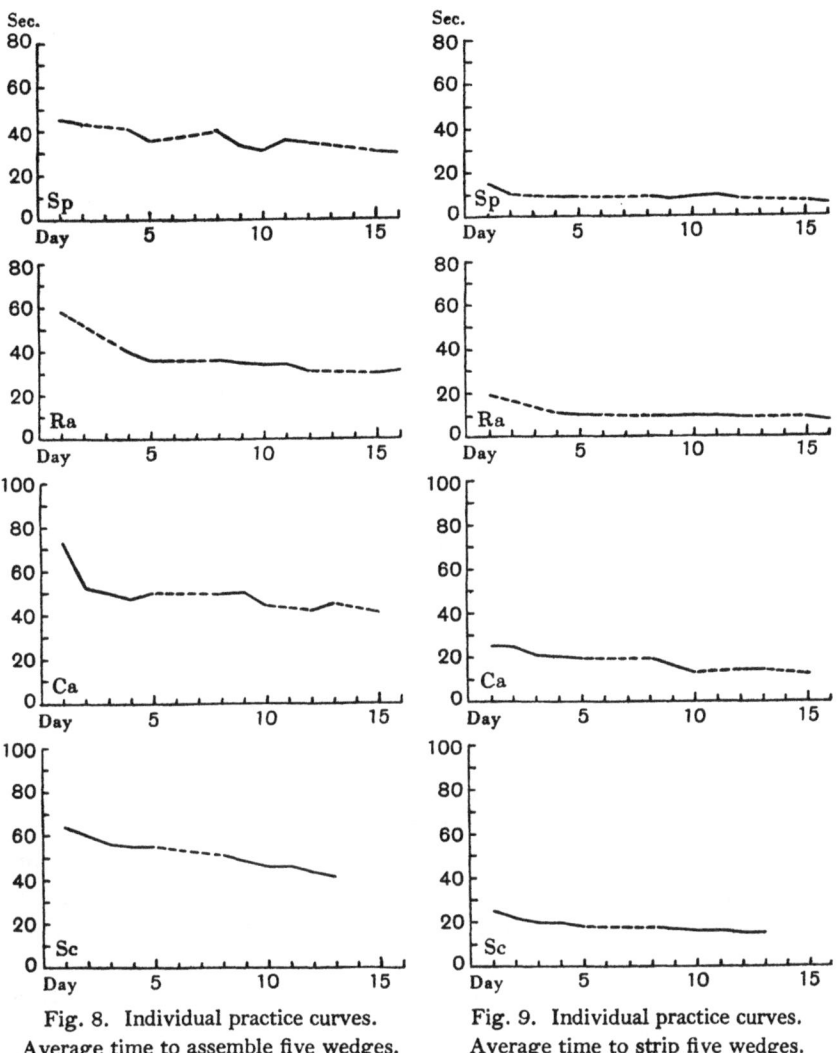

Fig. 8. Individual practice curves.
Average time to assemble five wedges.

Fig. 9. Individual practice curves.
Average time to strip five wedges.

(*d*) '*Wedges.*' Some individual curves of practice at assembling wedges are shown in fig. 8. The short steep 'initial' phase again makes its appearance in many of the curves.

Sp was the fastest subject on the total performance. He started second, dropped to fifth on the second and third practices, after which he rose to the first place which he closely maintained until the end. The course of improvement, although showing much irregularity, is seen to be fairly evenly spread throughout the practice period. In its absence of 'initial' phase and its almost straight line character (when smoothed out), the curve more resembles the type shown by Wi ('containers') and C ('porcelains') than by P ('porcelains') and Ra ('wedges')—all of whom were fast subjects. This subject was an amateur electrical engineer; and, as such, he had had much previous experience in the general handling of material, although he had not practised this particular operation. Consequently, the same explanation as seemed to account for the absence of the 'initial' phase in C (the writer) may account for it here—except that with C the previous training was in a sense 'theoretical', whereas here it is 'practical'. If so, we must suppose the 'cognitive' aspects which seems associated with the 'initial' phase to be more 'teachable' and 'transferable' than what, for lack of a better name, we have called the 'motor' aspect— a view which seems not unreasonable in the light of our analysis and of the results of our 'transfer' experiment.

Ra (fig. 8) was our second fastest subject on the whole performance, closely rivalling Sp (average time 36·8 sec. as against Sp's 36·7 sec.). His curve is much smoother throughout and shows a much greater rate of improvement initially. He made the greatest percentage improvement.

A similar difference in the distribution of progress appears in our two slowest subjects—Ca and Sc (fig. 8). The latter worked in stolid deliberate fashion, the former with evident haste and anxiety to beat his previous record. This dissimilarity may account for the difference in smoothness seen in the two curves. Ca showed the largest absolute improvement and the second largest percentage improvement. Sc ranked fourth for both. The second largest absolute improvement was shown by Wi, whose curve is not unlike that of Ca.

Four of our subjects had practised another operation some time before. In each case, the 'wedges' curves show some resemblance to the former curves.

Of the 'stripping' curves (fig. 9), the fastest for the whole performance are those of Sp and Ra (fig. 9). These subjects occupied the same rank (first and second respectively) as for the 'assembling' operation.

The slowest are again Sc and Ca (fig. 9), who also occupied the same ranks as in 'assembling'. Those of Ra and Sc are remarkably like their 'assembling' curves, especially when allowance is made for differences in the times of the two operations.[1] Sp's shows a steeper incline initially, but is otherwise not unlike his 'assembling' curve. In Ca's, the initial period of little progress and the 'steps', which have already appeared in other weak subjects, make their appearance, and the steep initial phase seen in his 'assembling' curve (and which is throughout more evident in the 'assembling' operations) is absent. The irregular character of Wi's 'assembling' curve is reproduced in her 'stripping' curve and she again makes her best score some time before practice terminates. While marked differences exist between individuals, the 'stripping' curve is thus seen to bear some similarity to the 'assembling' curve of the same individual.

(*e*) *General observations*. The following general observations arise out of the examination of the individual curves. They will, in some cases, be more evident from figs. 10 and 11.

(i) There are wide individual differences in all operations. These tend to diminish as practice continues. This tendency to draw closer together is more rapid in the early stages of practice and greater in the more complex operations such as those in assembling porcelains. It also continues longer for these processes and is augmented when greater complexity is introduced into the operation (cf. 'assembling' with 'stripping' in figs. 10 and 11).

(ii) The general course of progress seems much the same for most individuals, viz. continually less rapid as practice proceeds; but marked individual differences in speed and duration appear, and departures are sometimes observed—more especially in the simpler 'stripping' operations and the 'motor' phase of the 'assembling' operations—where the curve approximates closely to an oblique straight line. Where the operations are more complex (in the sense defined in Part IV) the practice curve is usually divisible into (*a*) an initial phase of steep slope followed by (*b*) a second phase of much more gradual slope. Exceptions appear in particularly weak subjects, where the transition from one phase to the other becomes less abrupt, and in those who are exceptionally good, where the initial phase tends to disappear.

[1] The unit of work on which the improvement is recorded is of much shorter duration in 'stripping'.

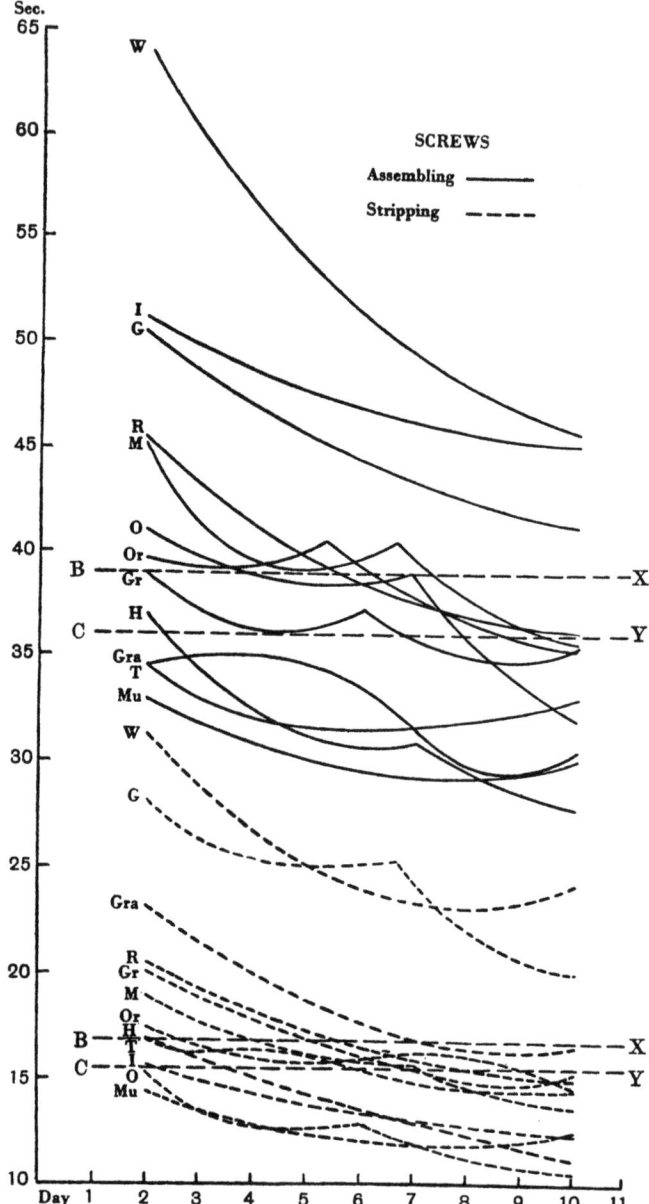

Fig. 10. Smoothed individual curves of practice at screws.
100 repetitions daily, in groups of ten. Average time for ten.

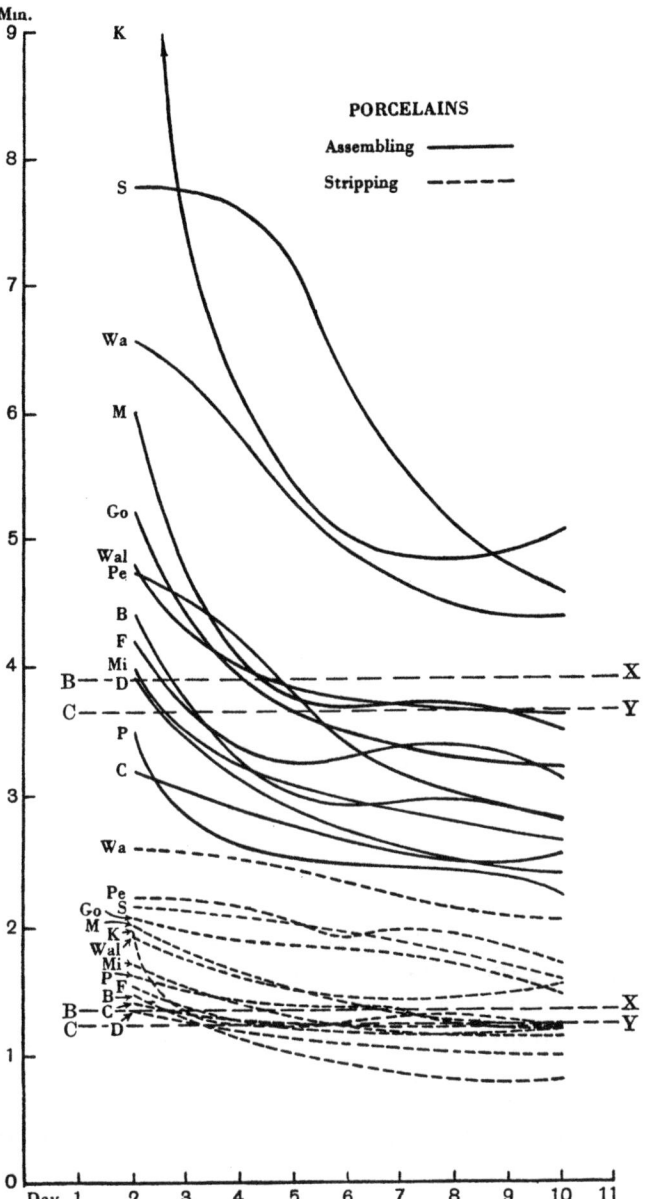

Fig. 11. Smoothed individual curves of practice at porcelains.
Twenty repetitions daily, in groups of five. Average time for five.

(iii) There are well-marked individual differences in the smoothness —or daily variability—shown in the curves. These are especially noticeable in the more complex of the operations. The jaggedness is sometimes confined to one part of the curve, but more frequently appears as a general character running throughout. Marked variability tends to be associated with weak ability.

2. Composite curves.

(*a*) *Preliminary considerations.* The individual curves may be combined into a composite curve by averaging the individual scores made on each day of practice. The curves so obtained are given in figs. 12–15.[1] The individual curves indicate features characteristic of the *individual*; these, by averaging out individual variations, bring out more clearly what is especially characteristic of the *operation*. They also show the course of progress for the group as a whole—often a more important consideration than the output of the individual.

In comparing the curves, it must be remembered that the shape will depend on (*a*) the unit of work taken as the basis for calculating ability at each practice, and (*b*) the amount of practice. With regard to (*a*), the unit taken in the present curves is the average time required to do a given quantity of work. In all except the 'screws' operation this consists in the 'assembling' or 'stripping' of five objects, i.e. five repetitions of the operation. For the much shorter 'screws' the unit taken is ten repetitions. This unit we have called a 'trial'. Since the number of trials which constituted a day's 'practice' at 'assembling' a given object was the same as at 'stripping' it and remained constant from day to day, the shapes of these respective curves *for that object* (i.e. in any one of the figs. 12–15) would remain unchanged had we taken as our unit the total time for the day's practice; for this merely means multiplying the times shown on the vertical scale by the number of 'trials' constituting a 'practice'. But the number of trials per practice for one object was not always the same as for another. This number is given in each figure. The details of the practice have been given in Chapter III.

Since the 'stripping' operation invariably occupied less time than 'assembling' and each operation was practised the same number of times, the amount of practice put in daily at the former was consider-

---

[1] These curves are obtained by averaging the actual scores of individual subjects. They have not been smoothed.

ably less, measured in terms of time, than that put in at the latter; and it diminished in both operations as practice continued. The actual times taken for a 'trial' on any day can be read directly from the graph. This multiplied by the number of trials gives the duration of practice for that day.

Before looking at the curves, one further observation may be worth making. So far, we have treated the 'assembling' and 'stripping' of the same object as two distinct operations. The same subject practised both on each occasion. It remains, therefore, a question as to how far practice at one may have influenced the other. Since both operations were practised together, any such influence should tend to be mutual and our results (described later) have disclosed no evidence that the effects of practising[1] one operation transfer to another. The introspections hint nowhere at the two operations interfering with one another. On the whole, then, it seems unlikely that any serious change in the shape of the curve was introduced by practising the complementary operation. At the same time, the fact that both 'assembling' and 'stripping' were practised together must be recognized; they really constitute two parts of a single 'practised' operation.

(b) *The 'assembling' curves.* With these considerations in mind, we now turn to the curves themselves, confining attention first to the assembling operations.

Perhaps the most striking feature of the assembling curve for 'screws' (fig. 12) is its remarkable smoothness over the first seven practices. The irregularity seen in the last three days may be merely an expression of the tendency for the individual to display greater variation from day to day as the limits of improvement are reached. Such variations could hardly be expected to smooth out in so small a group. The rise on the last day of practice may have been partly due to the week-end rest which, for most subjects, immediately preceded this, or to the 'Monday' effect. Even so, it would only provide another example of variable influences becoming more evident as the limits of practice are reached.

If this rise in the curve be discounted for the reasons just given, an alternative explanation is possible, viz. that as the limits of practice are approached 'plateaux' are more likely to appear. On this view, the last three days are not so much indicative of irregularity as of a plateau on the ninth and tenth days. If so, further improvement would

---

[1] As distinguished from 'training', see Chapter XIII.

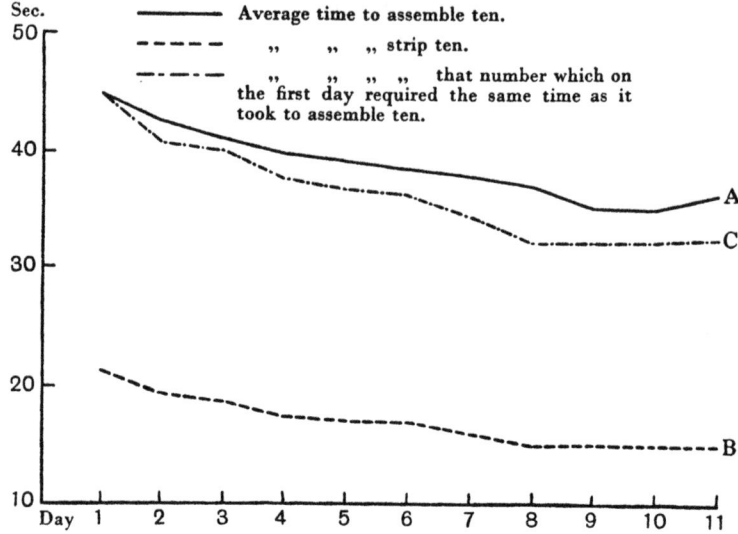

Fig. 12. Composite practice curves of twelve adults.
A day's practice = 100 repetitions in groups of ten.

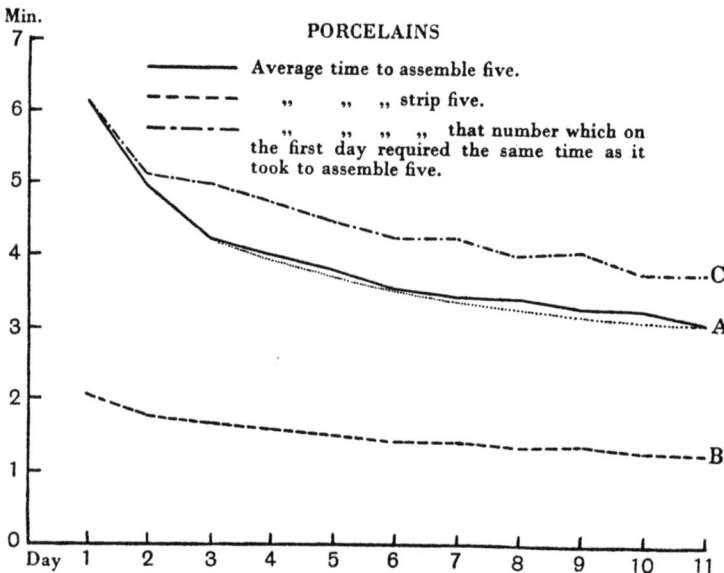

Fig. 13. Composite practice curves of thirteen adults.
A day's practice = twenty repetitions in groups of five.

be expected to take the course of relatively sharp falls (as shown on the ninth day) alternating with plateaux. Examples of such plateaux towards the end of the curve appear in fig. 13 (*A*) on the ninth and tenth days, and in fig. 14 (*A*) on the seventh and eighth days.

In *A* of fig. 13 we have the curve of the longest and most complex of the operations. It is also the steepest of the assembling curves—

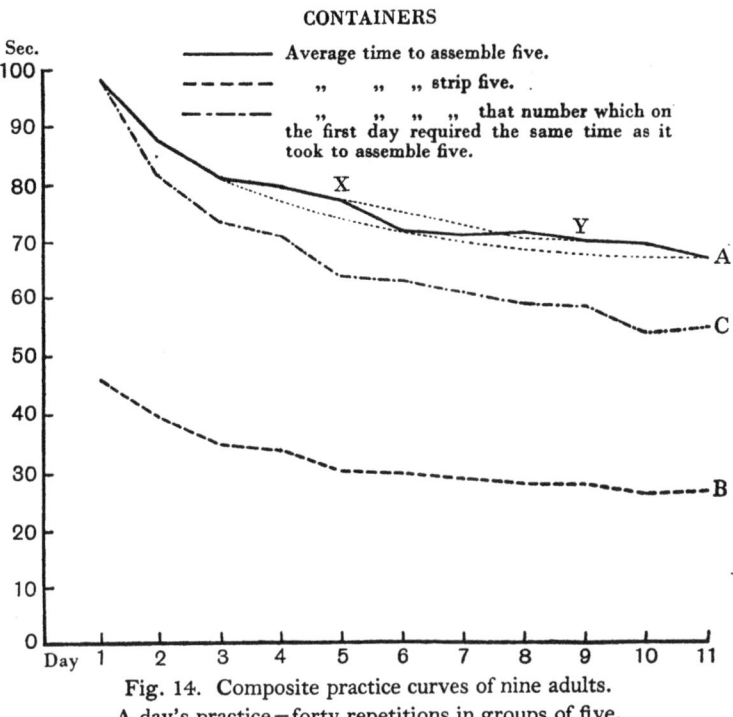

CONTAINERS

Fig. 14. Composite practice curves of nine adults.
A day's practice = forty repetitions in groups of five.

showing the greatest improvement both in the 'absolute' sense and also when the gain is measured as a percentage of the time taken to effect the operation (49 per cent.). In this respect, it contrasts strongly with the curve of the simplest operation which we have just examined. In shape it falls into three approximately straight lines, viz. an initial line of steep descent from the first to the third day of practice, a less steep line from the third to the sixth day, followed by one of still more gradual slope which continues up to the last day. The first of these represents the 'initial' phase—less clearly defined here than in the individual curves owing to the smoothing effect of combining these curves.

The curve for assembling 'containers' (shown in *A* of fig. 14) bears a remarkable resemblance to that for porcelains in forming three sections which approximate to straight lines rather than to a single curve. But its general descent is seen to be less steep than the 'porcelain' curve when the total improvement shown is considered as a percentage of the time taken initially (32·7 per cent.), and is, of course, much less so when measured in absolute units of time; and the 'initial' phase is less clearly distinguishable. This accords with the individual curves and with the analysis given in Part IV.

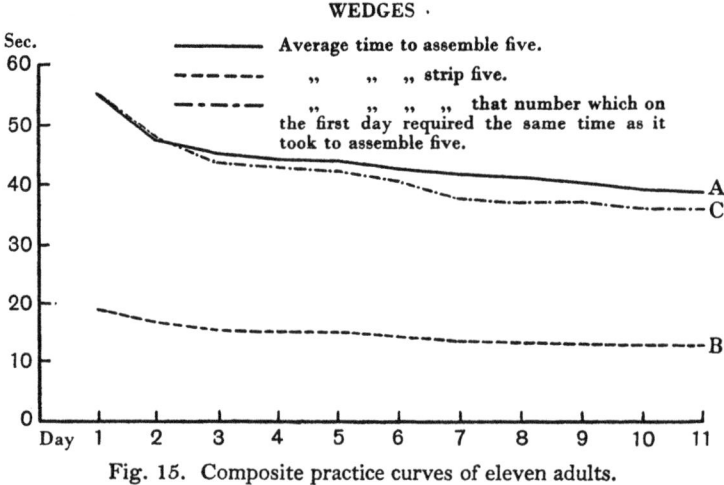

Fig. 15. Composite practice curves of eleven adults.
A day's practice = fifty repetitions in groups of five.

A of fig. 15 is the curve for assembling 'wedges'. It, too, divides into three parts which differ in slope in similar fashion to the porcelain and container curves—the points of division being at the second and third days. In this less complex operation, the first two parts—the periods of most rapid improvement—are seen to be of shorter duration than in the two preceding curves. The initial phase is clearly distinguishable from the succeeding phase of more gradual descent which follows after the second day of practice and which, we have suggested, seems more closely associated with the motor aspect of the operation. This part of the curve bears a close resemblance to the 'screws' curve shown in fig. 12 (*A*), i.e. to another operation in which the movements are simple in character. The absence of the steep 'initial' phase in the screws curve and its presence in the curve for wedges agree with the fact that the processes associated with this phase play a much larger part in the wedges operation.

Before leaving the assembling curves it may be observed that, in figs. 13 and 14, the points of junction of the three sections into which these curves divide lie on a curve (shown by the dotted line) which resembles the shape commonly associated with the curve of practice at mental work. This tendency for parts of the curve to flatten into a straight line, or even to assume a convex form, is also to be seen in the other composite curves and in very many of the individual curves. It is interesting to speculate whether this is a distinguishing feature of 'motor' learning.[1]

(c) *The 'stripping' curves.* The points of main interest in the stripping curves are similar to those which we have already examined in the assembling curves. In each case, the stripping curve bears a close resemblance in its general course to the corresponding assembling curve. The chief points of difference are their less steep gradients and their less clearly defined 'initial' phase—features which we have already had occasion to associate with the longer and more complex assembling operations. The less complex operations (screws and wedges) are again seen to yield the smoother and less steeply inclined curves.

So far, we have used such terms as 'gradient' and 'smoothness' in the absolute sense, i.e. as indicated by the absolute gain in time shown directly in the curve. When one curve is compared with another, the considerations with which this section opened must be kept in mind; namely that the operations varied with respect to the time taken by a 'trial' and a 'practice'. The condition common to both assembling and stripping curves in any one figure is the number of repetitions of the operation which constituted a trial and the number of trials to a practice. Since a trial at stripping was invariably shorter than one at assembling, the absolute improvement shown in the stripping curves was effected on a unit of work (a 'trial') and by an amount of practice which occupied less time than was the case in the corresponding assembling curve. For example, in fig. 12 curve *B*, the reduction on the second day of 1·7 sec. was made on a trial which took only 21 sec. to strip on the first day, whereas the reduction of 2·5 sec. seen on the

---

[1] A similar feature is observable in many of the curves of practice obtained by Dr J. C. Flügel at work which involved addition and writing. See his *Practice, Fatigue and Oscillation* (Camb. Univ. Press).

same day in curve *A* was made on a trial (comprising the same number of repetitions) which required as much as 45 sec. on the first day.

To show more closely the times required to assemble and to strip amounts which initially took equal times, we have plotted curve *C*. Thus in fig. 12 this shows the time taken each day to strip that number of screws (21·4) which took on the first day the same time (45 sec.) as a single trial at assembling this material; and similarly as regards figs. 13–15. It should be noted that the times for curve *C* are not merely theoretical derivations from *B* but were the actual average daily times for this quantity of stripping; also that by thus equalizing the times the number of repetitions at stripping represented by the points on curve *C* now far exceeds that at assembling, and that the total time spent at practice remains, as before, greater for assembling than for stripping and to the extent shown by direct comparison of curves *A* and *B*.

The chief interest of the *C* curves lies in the observation that in three cases the stripping curves are thus seen to have a steeper gradient than the assembling curves. The exception occurs in the most complex of the operations and one in which the 'initial' phase is most marked, viz. that of assembling porcelains. This means that the rate of improvement, when expressed as a percentage of the time taken to do the work, is greater in the simpler stripping operations. It may be inferred that under conditions of equal lengths of practice the stripping operations would have shown a still greater advance in percentage improvement.

Taken in conjunction with the *B* curves, the results suggest that when practised an equal number of times[1] the more complex operation, up to a certain degree of complexity, will show the greater absolute gain but the smaller percentage gain, and that as this degree of complexity is exceeded the more complex operation tends to show the greater gain both in the absolute and in the relative sense.

3. 'INITIAL' AND 'TERMINAL' ABILITY CURVES.

It will be remembered that each of our subjects was tested at the various operations before undergoing practice. Fig. 16 gives the average performance of all our subjects at each of the five successive trials which constituted the initial test. A trial here, in all except the screws operations, consists of a single assemblage and is, therefore, not

---

[1] Under the same general conditions as obtained in the research.

to be confused with the longer trials referred to in the curves of the practice period.

A 'practice' effect is clearly evident in these initial tests—particularly

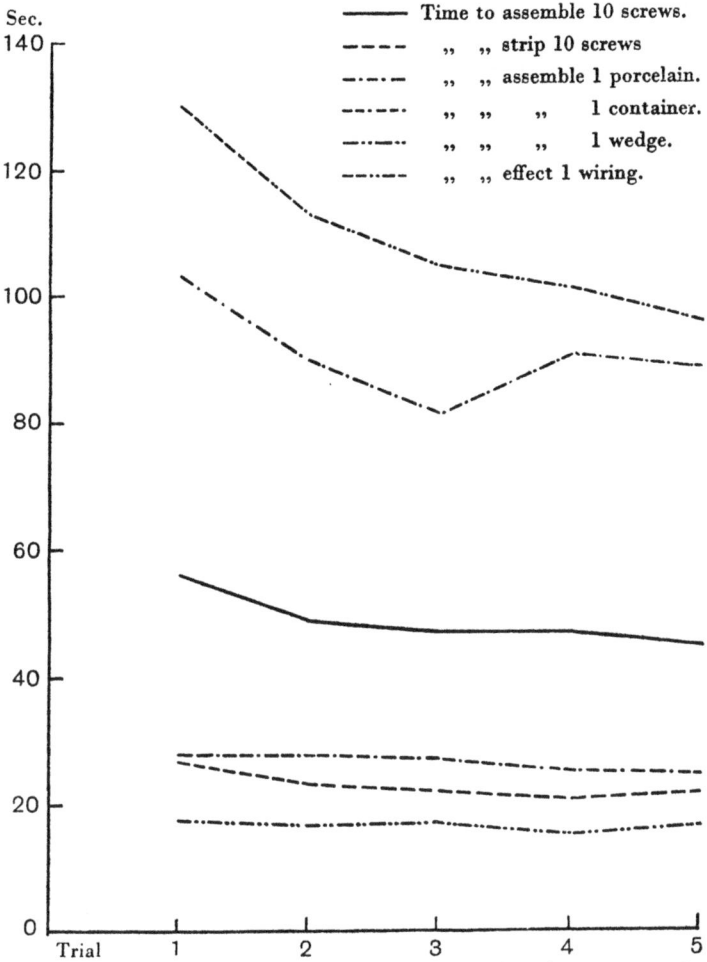

Fig. 16. Composite curves of fifty adults, showing the scores at the five successive 'trials' which constituted the measure of initial ability at the routine assembling operations.

in the two longest and most complex operations (wiring and porcelains) and in the two (assembling and stripping screws) where the increased number of repetitions to the 'trial' afforded greater practice. The general tendency for improvement to become less rapid as practice continues, which appeared in the curves of longer practice, is also seen to hold of these very short trials; and similar differences in gradient as between long and short operations again appear. The steeper fall of the stripping curve for screws as compared with the assembling curve for containers suggests that the observations which arose out of the comparison of curves *A* and *C* in figs. 12–15 also apply to the very limited practice afforded here—for a trial at the screws occupied approximately the same time as a trial at the much more complex containers, but comprised ten times the number of repetitions.

The indications of fatigue, seen in the upward turn taken by the porcelains curve on the fourth trial, are interesting in view of the absence of any general awareness of fatigue by the subjects. It was, however, the operation most likely to induce fatigue. Signs of fatigue also appear in the last trial at wedges and at stripping screws.

In the right-hand halves of figs. 25 and 26 we have under 'terminal ability' the scores made on repeating these tests under similar conditions after the period of practice (at other tests) or of rest (in the case of 'controls') had intervened. They represent the subject's second attempt at the tests. Apart from the greater irregularities to be expected from smaller groups, and the somewhat lower gradient consistent with a later stage of practice, they show the same general feature as in the initial tests. Perhaps the most interesting fact is the tendency for the curves in the second testing to go on roughly from where they leave off in the first, notwithstanding that over a fortnight intervened between the two.

B. PRACTICE CURVES OF SCHOOLBOYS

1. INDIVIDUAL CURVES.

Some of the curves of practice for the five-day period carried out by our schoolboys, selected from different parts of the scale of ability, are shown in figs. 17–20.[1] Individual differences similar to those to which attention has already been directed in the adult curves reappear in these,—in particular the more jagged shape of the curves in weaker subjects, their steeper fall initially (except in those subjects like Gr and Ov (fig. 19), who appear to have had great difficulty in surmounting this initial 'cognitive' phase), and their greater absolute improvement.

[1] For 'screws' and 'porcelains' only; see footnote to p. 49. Our observations in this section are based on the whole of the curves, not merely on those which it has been possible to show here.

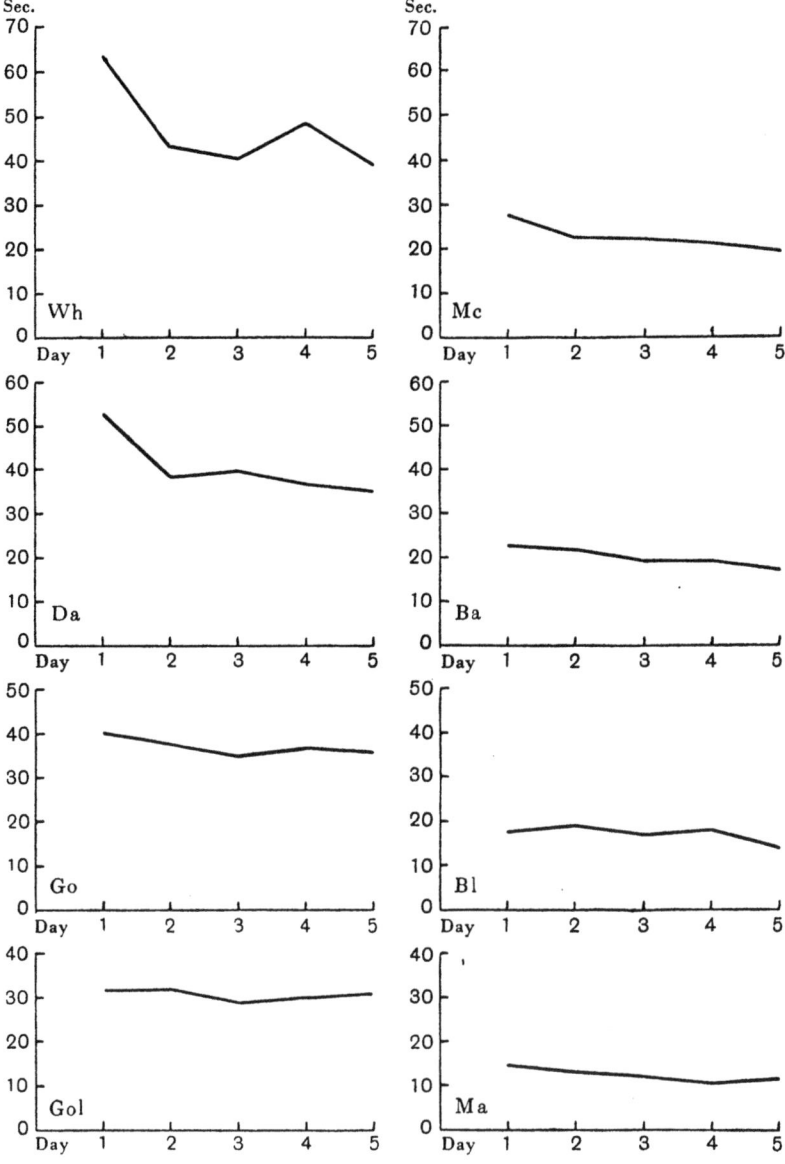

Fig. 17. Individual practice curves.
Average time to assemble ten screws.
Eighty repetitions daily, in groups
of twenty.

Fig. 18. Individual practice curves.
Average time to strip ten screws.
Eighty repetitions daily, in groups
of twenty.

These individual characteristics are best seen by a glance at the curves themselves, and it would be hardly profitable to describe them in detail. The curves of Gr are, however, noteworthy. The irregularity of his assembling curves are in conformity with the extremely weak 'initial' phase already noticed in certain of the adult subjects. He seems never to have mastered the processes associated with this initial phase. It represents a genuine disability; for this subject, whom we knew personally, was undoubtedly anxious to do well. As the practice continued, a further handicap appeared in the evident distress he felt at being by far the slowest of his group. He also started badly in the stripping operations, where, it will be remembered, the finer movements involved in the adjustment of one part to another were largely absent; but here he shows a decided improvement with practice. In the simpler of these operations (fig. 20), his curve is fairly smooth, but much irregularity occurs in the curve of the more complex container operation.

The assembling curve of Ov (fig. 19)—another very weak subject —contrasts strongly with that of Gr in its regular and rapid descent after the initial difficulties had been overcome in the first two practices. In assembling containers he does not differ so markedly from the other subjects, although he again ranks very low and makes no progress after the third practice. Reference to his stripping curves (shown for porcelains in fig. 20) shows him to be equally weak at these operations and equally lacking in progress.

On comparing the individual curves with each other, it is seen that although a fair amount of overlapping occurs as the practice continues, there is observable an underlying tendency for the subjects to retain their initial positions. This tendency for 'ability' on one day to correlate with 'ability' on another appears more marked in the simpler operations. The greater number of repetitions per practice which these operations permitted, with a consequently more exhaustive and reliable measure of 'ability' on each occasion, may partly account for this.

Generally speaking, the curves are more irregular, and in many cases indicate a less rapid and less continuous improvement than is shown in the 'adult' subjects. Several causes would operate in this direction—the greater variability of reaction to be expected of children, the shorter daily practice, and the previously mentioned tendency for more haste to result often in less speed. Undue haste of this kind

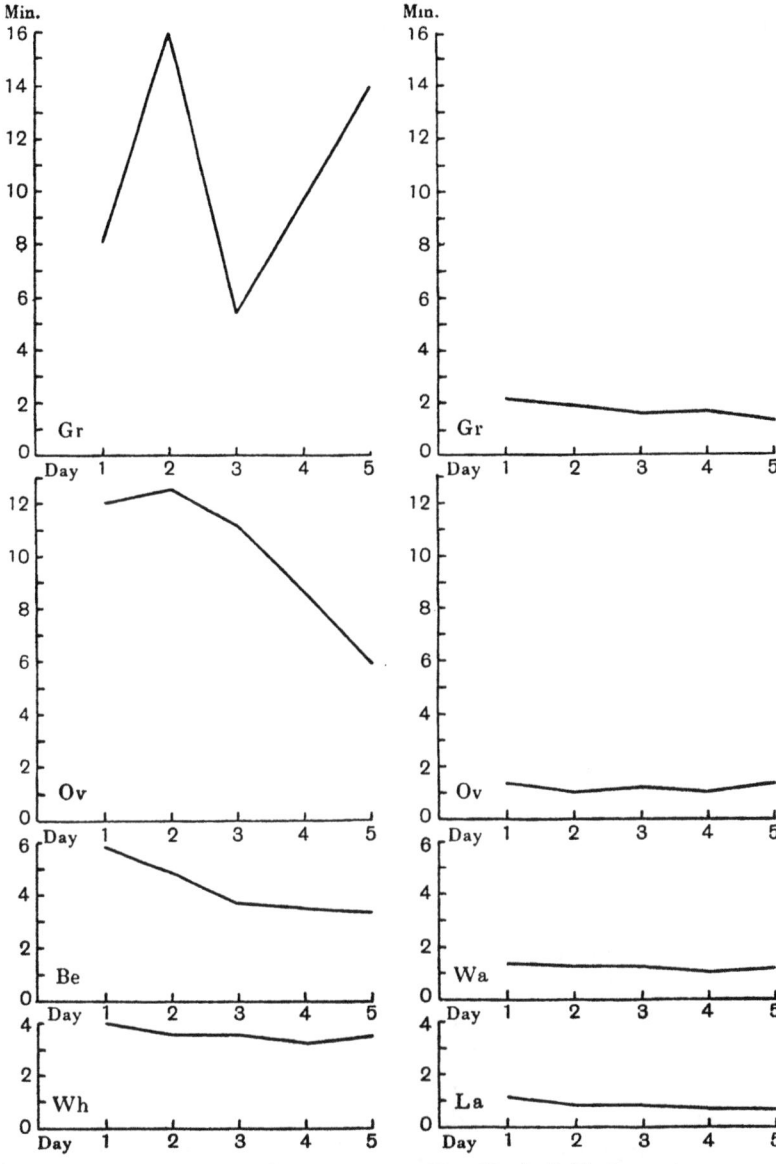

Fig. 19. Individual practice curves. Average time to assemble five porcelains. Ten repetitions daily, in groups of five.

Fig. 20. Individual practice curves. Average time to strip five porcelains. Ten repetitions daily, in groups of five.

—rather than any lack of interest—seems to account for the rise seen in some of these curves towards the end of the week, i.e. as it became increasingly difficult to improve on the score.[1] In 'screws' and 'containers' a probable cause of the slower progress shown by the schoolboys was their greater ability at first, for we have seen that initial ability correlates inversely with improvability. These group differences are best seen in the composite curves to which we now turn.

2. COMPOSITE CURVES.

(*a*) '*Assembling*' *compared with* '*stripping*'. The composite curves are shown in figs. 21–24. Comparison between the assembling and the stripping curves (*A* and *B*) indicates a difference similar to that already observed in the curves of our 'adult' group, viz. that improvement in the absolute time to effect the operation is greater and more rapid in the more complex operations, and especially so during the initial phase of these operations.

The *C* curves show, as before, the daily times to effect that number of stripping operations which on the first day took the same time as the assembling work represented in curve *A*. Comparison between these curves as regards their relative steepness shows agreement with the adult group in the simplest (screws) and the most complex (porcelain) operations. Thus *C* is steeper than *A* in the first, and conversely so in the latter. But in those of intermediate complexity ('wedges' and 'containers') the relationship seen in the adult curves is reversed in the boys' curves, for in these operations the assembling curve (*A*) is steeper than the stripping curve (*C*)—a condition only seen in the very complex porcelain test with adults.

This difference between the groups might be explained by supposing that the difference in complexity as between assembling and stripping is greater in the younger subjects than it is in the more developed adult group, so that in the boys the assembling operation shows more rapid progress than the stripping operation, not only in the case of the most complex, porcelain, material (as with adults), but also in the less complex 'wedges' and 'containers'. If so, this developmental difference would seem to be associated with those processes which call for the careful and accurate adjustment of parts and of forces rather than for mere speed of movement; because in the simple

---

[1] It will be remembered that the number of times the best previous score was improved on determined, in part, the award of prizes.

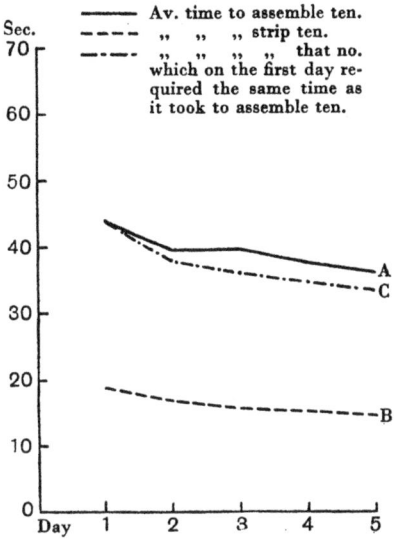

SCREWS

Av. time to assemble ten.
„ „ „ strip ten.
„ „ „ „ that no.
which on the first day required the same time as
it took to assemble ten.

Fig. 21. Composite practice curves of
twenty boys.

A day's practice = eighty repetitions
in groups of twenty.

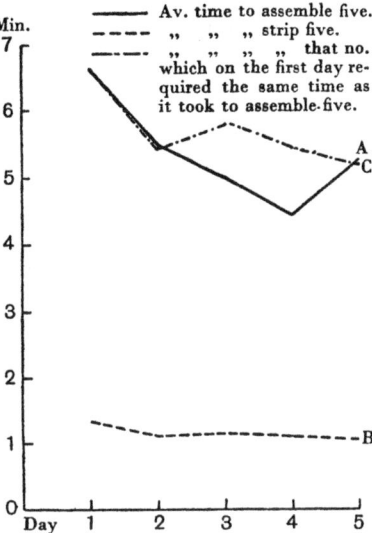

PORCELAINS

Av. time to assemble five.
„ „ „ strip five.
„ „ „ „ that no.
which on the first day required the same time as
it took to assemble five.

Fig. 22. Composite practice curves of
sixteen boys.

A day's practice = ten repetitions in
groups of five.

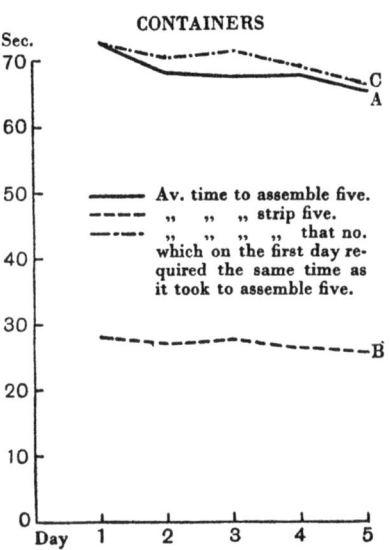

CONTAINERS

Av. time to assemble five.
„ „ „ strip five.
„ „ „ „ that no.
which on the first day required the same time as
it took to assemble five.

Fig. 23. Composite practice curves of
twenty boys.

A day's practice = thirty repetitions in
groups of five.

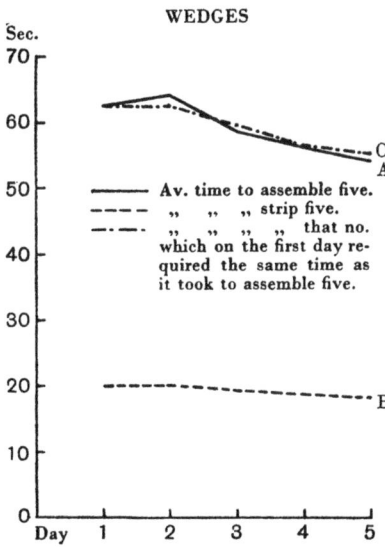

WEDGES

Av. time to assemble five.
„ „ „ strip five.
„ „ „ „ that no.
which on the first day required the same time as
it took to assemble five.

Fig. 24. Composite practice curves of
twenty boys.

A day's practice = thirty repetitions in
groups of five.

operations of assembling and stripping 'screws', the boys are superior both in the time taken to effect the operation and in the amount of progress shown.

But, while a developmental factor of this kind may have played a part, an examination of the actual times taken and of the amount of improvement shown suggests an alternative explanation based on the difference in the conditions of practice for the two groups and in the differences in initial ability. Here, however, we are on less secure ground, since the precise effect of a change in these conditions and of a simultaneous change in mental development is unknown, whereas we do know that the conditions for 'assembling' were the same as those for 'stripping' within the same group—which is all that the above explanation supposes.

Examining this alternative explanation in the case of 'wedges' (figs. 15 and 24), we see that the adult curve falls about as much in two days as the boys' curve falls in the whole five (approximately 8 sec.). If, on this account, we regard the whole of the boys' curve as representing the same phase of learning as is represented by the first two days in the adults', the difference between the two groups as regards the relative steepness of A and C disappears; for, in this part of the adult curve, C is seen to be related to A in much the same way as it is throughout the whole of the boys' curve.

In the container operations (figs. 14 and 23), this method of comparison is not applicable, since the fall in the boys' curve for the whole week is less than that which occurs on the second day with the adults. This would seem largely due to the much greater initial ability with which the boys start, for initial ability, as will be seen in Chapter xii, is inversely correlated with improvability. We can, however, choose a section on the adult assembling curve over which approximately the same amount of improvement is shown as occurs from the beginning to the end of the boys' assembling curve. Such a section is XY. If we now compare the corresponding section of the stripping curve (B) with the boys' stripping curve, the two are seen to show closely similar amounts of improvement (approximately 2·75 sec.). The dotted line joining XY on curve A (fig. 14) shows this part of curve B corresponding to C of fig. 23. This means that when the absolute amounts of improvement are taken into account, there is little difference between the two groups as regards relationship between the progress made in 'assembling' and that made at 'stripping'.

(b) '*Ability*' and '*improvability*' *compared with adults.* This does not dispose of the differences observable in the progress itself. Thus, in both of the simple screws operations, the boys begin better than the adults and show greater improvement over the five days' practice, in spite of their daily practice being only 80 per cent. of the work done by the adults.

Comparison in the case of the 'porcelain' assembling operation is complicated owing to the difference in the daily amounts of practice done by the two groups. The adults' average is better for the first day, but this represents the average of trials[1] 2–5 (the first trial being the initial test), whereas in the boys it is the average of trials 3 and 4. Similarly, on the second day the adults' figure represents the average of trials 6–9, the boys' trials 5 and 6. By the end of the third day (average of trials 7 and 8), the boys had assembled forty porcelains, i.e. five less than the adults had assembled by the end of the second day. The time for the boys on the third day (5 min.) is only a few seconds less than that for the adults on the second, and they had slightly less practice. On the next day (fourth) the boys improve by approximately 35 sec. through practising the operation ten times, while the adults (third day) showed an improvement of approximately 42 sec. through a practice of twice this length. When, therefore, allowance is made for the difference in practice, there seems little to choose between the groups.[2]

But with 'wedges' the adults are superior in ability throughout. Thus, in the assembling operations, they started quicker by 7 sec. per trial (after less practice) and reached a speed which was only just exceeded by the boys on the last day; and similar remarks apply to stripping, except that the difference was not so great for this shorter operation. A like consideration also applies to 'improvability'; for the gain of approximately 8 sec. made by the adults on the second day, as the result of fifty additional repetitions of the operation, was only equalled by the boys on the last day, after 120 additional repetitions.

The 'container' curves are not directly comparable, since this

---

[1] A trial consists in assembling five 'porcelains'.

[2] The rise in the boys' assembling curve on the fifth day is partly due to our very erratic subject Gr—but not entirely, since it also occurs when Gr is omitted. It may have been caused by a last day spurt engendering more haste than speed, or by the accumulated week's fatigue manifesting itself in this—the most complex and difficult operation. Owing to a change of procedure which greatly reduced the time, the boys' 'stripping' curve is not comparable with the adults.

operation was modified for the boys by the omission of one part—the assembly of the ring *C*. Here, too, as in the other operations (except 'screws'), allowance must be made for the longer test taken initially (i.e. before beginning the practice proper) by the boys—a fact which makes the first points on the boys' 'container' curves correspond more closely to a point mid-way between the first and second points on the adult curves. In the case of 'assembling', the faster times shown throughout in the boys' curves seem accounted for by these differences, but hardly so in 'stripping', where the figures suggest a superiority in the boys even after allowing for the difference in conditions.

Comparison of 'improvability' is also complicated by the difference in the lengths of daily practice.[1] But if, as before, we disregard for the moment the distribution of the repetitions and consider merely their number, we see that after the 120 repetitions of the 'assembling' operations which intervened between the first and last points on their curve the boys improve by approximately 8 sec. on an initial score of 73 sec. (per trial). This is equivalent to a gain of 9·5 sec. on a score of 87·5 sec.—the time taken by the adults on their second day when they were at approximately the same stage of practice.[2] Reference to the adult 'assembling' curve shows this group to improve by 8 sec. as a result of the 100 repetitions which intervened between the second and fourth points, and by 2·5 sec. as the result of a further fifty repetitions. This gives an estimated improvement of 9·25 sec. for 125 repetitions—a figure which closely approximates to the boys' 9·5 sec. for 120 repetitions. While this estimate is necessarily only a rough one, and ignores the difference in the daily distribution of the repetitions, it serves to indicate that the apparent differences in the curves offer no serious reason for supposing one group to be superior to the other, either in 'ability' or in 'improvability'. It is interesting to notice that even these apparent differences in shape largely disappear when it is remembered that the first point on the boys' curve corresponds more nearly to the practice stage reached on the second day by the adults.

In the case of the 'container' stripping operation, it is impossible to compare the curves as we have done above, since the difference in

---

[1] These modifications in the boys' data were rendered necessary by time and other considerations, for this comparison between the groups was not the primary aim of the work.
[2] The difference between 73 sec. and 87·5 sec. is regarded as approximately the additional time required to assemble the ring which was omitted from the boys' material. The estimate which follows also assumes that the simple additional act of assembling the ring would not greatly alter the shape of the boys' curve.

times between the groups is large enough to suggest a definite superiority, in at least the early stages, in favour of the boys. But, if we make the reasonable assumption that the shape of the curve was not seriously altered by the omission of the ring from the boys' material, we can estimate the approximate percentage improvement made for a given number of repetitions. Calculating as before, we find the boys make a gain of 2·08 per cent. as a result of 120 repetitions spread over five days, the adults gain 5·5 per cent. for 100 repetitions over three days, 6 per cent. for 150 repetitions over four days. Unless we suppose —contrary to general opinion—that the wider spread of practice acted adversely in the boys, these figures give a greater percentage improvability to the adults.

(*c*) *Summary*. To sum up the results of the last section, the curves indicate that under equal conditions of practice the boys, as a group, are of superior 'ability' and 'improvability' (both absolute and percentage) at the simpler operations of assembling and stripping 'screws'. Where, among the more complex operations, comparison is most direct, as in the assembling and stripping of 'wedges', the adults are superior in these respects. The varying conditions of practice in the case of the 'porcelain' and 'container' assembling operations render comparison difficult; but, so far as we can allow for these, the differences observed are not such as to suggest any important difference in 'ability' or 'improvability' between the groups. In the simpler work of 'stripping' containers the boys seem of superior ability but show less percentage improvability.

C. 'INITIAL' COMPARED WITH 'TERMINAL' ABILITY

1. ADULTS.

When using vocational tests it is of crucial importance to know how far ability at the test is indicative of the skill to which the testee may ultimately attain after practice at his work. Light on this may be shed by comparing the ability shown by our subjects on the first day of practice with that shown on the last. The correlations between the rank orders on these two days are as follows: for *assembling*, screws 0·66, porcelains 0·81, containers 0·69, wedges 0·53, and for *stripping*, screws 0·72, porcelains 0·90, containers 0·65, wedges 0·14. It is seen that in every operation except stripping wedges there is a fairly close correspondence between ability on the first day and that on the last day. Owing to the small size of the groups, too much importance must not be placed on the absolute values of the coefficients. They provide the best means of expressing, in simple fashion, the extent of the agreement between the order of merit on the first day and that on the last.

In making this comparison, it must be remembered that the measures of ability are not of perfect reliability, i.e. a rank order at the test would not agree perfectly with a second rank order made at the same sitting, and that as subjects approach one another in ability it becomes harder to assign their true order of merit. This seems to account for the low agreement seen in stripping wedges, where the whole range of ability tested extends over only some 10 sec. per trial and about one-half of the subjects are grouped very closely together.

2. SCHOOLBOYS.

A similar correspondence between initial and terminal ability was found with our larger schoolboy groups. The correlations between ability on the first day and that on the last (fifth) are, for the assembling operations, screws 0·81, wedges 0·55, porcelains 0·56, containers 0·58, and for stripping, 0·66, 0·76, 0·17, and 0·45, respectively.

Reference to p. 44 shows that, with one exception, these figures are of the same order as the reliability coefficients, so that, on the whole, the tests predict future ability (after practice) to about the same degree of accuracy as they measure 'present' ability.

CHAPTER XI

THE TRANSFER OF 'PRACTICE' EFFECTS

A. INTRODUCTORY

Having examined the more important effects of practice on 'ability', we have now to consider how these are related to other functions, confining our attention first to the question of 'transfer'—namely whether the improvement effected by *practising* one operation transfers to other operations. We shall reserve for later consideration the analogous question with respect to conditions of *training*.[1]

The practical bearing of this question has already been remarked on in Chapter II, as relating to the problem of transferring workers from one operation to another. Sometimes there is a choice of operations from which workers may be transferred, as often happens where there is a seasonal demand for certain goods. There the practical application goes beyond the general question as to whether transfer occurs at all, to the special question as to where, among the various operations, transfer will operate most effectively. By examining the transfer effects of practice at a variety of operations it was hoped to throw light on the general conditions which govern any 'transfer' that might be found.

Mention has also been made already of the bearing of this question on schemes of manual training. In devising such courses it is clearly important to know how far an intensive training which aims at the attainment of great skill at a relatively restricted group of activities is to be preferred to a more general training in a greater variety of operations. The answer to such a question must, of course, depend on a number of considerations, including the aim of the course. Of these, an important one must frequently be whether the skill developed in the course will transfer to other operations. Here, again, it was thought that the comparative study of the transfer effects of various kinds of practice might have a fruitful bearing on such questions as the grouping of subjects in the curriculum, and the grouping of operations in the workshop or assembling room.

[1] See p. 21 and Chapter XIII.

The question is not without its theoretical interest. If 'transfer' were found to occur between operations which had, initially, nothing in common, it would suggest that the processes involved in learning to acquire greater skill are different from those which come specifically into play in carrying out the operation. If, again, transfer occurred only between operations highly saturated with the 'routine' factor, it would suggest that the processes underlying the transferred improvement are the same as those which determine 'ability' itself. If, as a third alternative, there were found no transfer of practice effects, the processes which had been speeded up or changed, as the result of practice in one operation, can hardly be the same as those upon which the acquisition of further skill in the other depends; nor can the improvement be associated with a change in the common 'routine' factor. This latter alternative is, indeed, the one found in our results.

B. DATA FROM ADULT GROUPS

It will be remembered that our adult subjects, after being tested for 'initial' ability on six operations, were assigned to one of five groups. Four of these groups practised, respectively, one of four operations selected from these six—the practice consisting of the double operation of alternately assembling and stripping the material—while the fifth—a 'control' group—refrained from any special practice at motor operations. At the end of this period, all were re-tested for 'terminal' ability at each of the six operations.

Charts similar to figs. 25 and 26 have been drawn up for each practised group.[1] In the left-hand column of these are given the initial measures of practisers and controls at all six operations, and in the right-hand column the terminal measures. The five points on each curve show the times for each of the five trials which constituted the measure.[2]

On comparing practisers with controls we find, in the case of all four practised groups, that although the practised subjects usually show some improvement in their terminal scores at the unpractised operations it is nowhere clearly greater than that shown by the control group. This improvement is therefore to be attributed to the practice

[1] See footnote to p. 49.
[2] Here a 'trial' consisted of a single assemblage of the material, except in the case of assembling and stripping screws, where ten repetitions of the operation constituted a 'trial'.

afforded by the second (terminal) testing of the unpractised operation itself rather than to any transfer from the practised operation. More often than not the terminal curve continues from where the initial curve leaves off, as if no period of time—much less of practice at another operation—had intervened.[1]

The extension of our investigation over four practised operations meant a corresponding reduction in the size of our groups. We may,

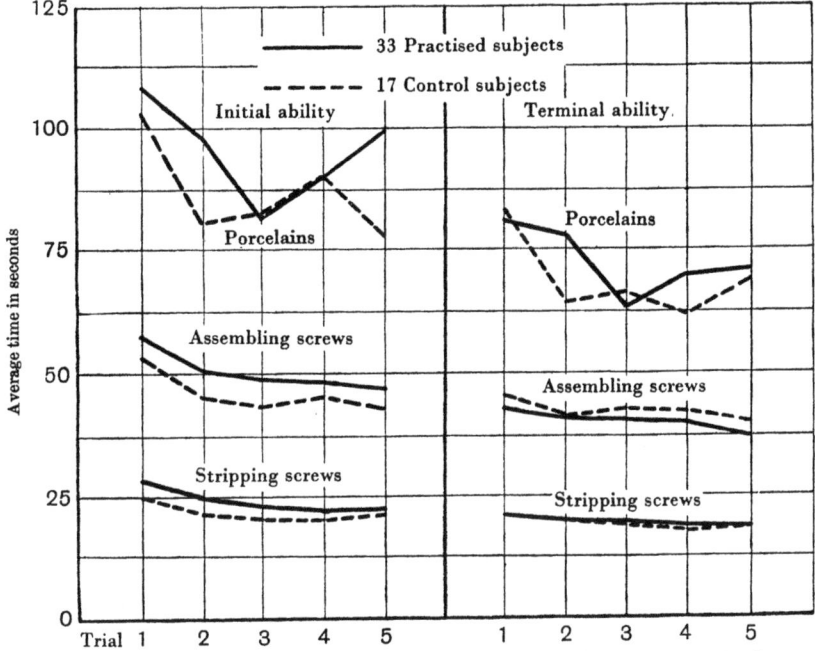

Fig. 25. Comparison between initial and terminal abilities of practised and control groups.

however, combine (by averaging) the initial measures of all operations, and the terminal measures of the unpractised operations, for the whole of the practised groups. We thus obtain initial and terminal measures of a much larger group, all of whom had practised, in the meantime, some other operation than that for which they were terminally measured. Owing to the larger size of the group, any indications of 'transfer' will now have greater statistical significance.

[1] The terminal scores of the practised operation invariably show marked improvement over the initial scores, leaving no doubt about the existence of a practice effect much in excess of that shown in the unpractised operations.

These initial and terminal measures, derived now from thirty-three practised subjects, are given in figs. 25 and 26, where it will be seen that the initial and terminal curves fall in approximately the same positions on the chart as do those of the control group. At first sight, a slight transfer effect is suggested by the curves of (i) assembling screws and (ii) assembling wedges; but, in both cases, the observed

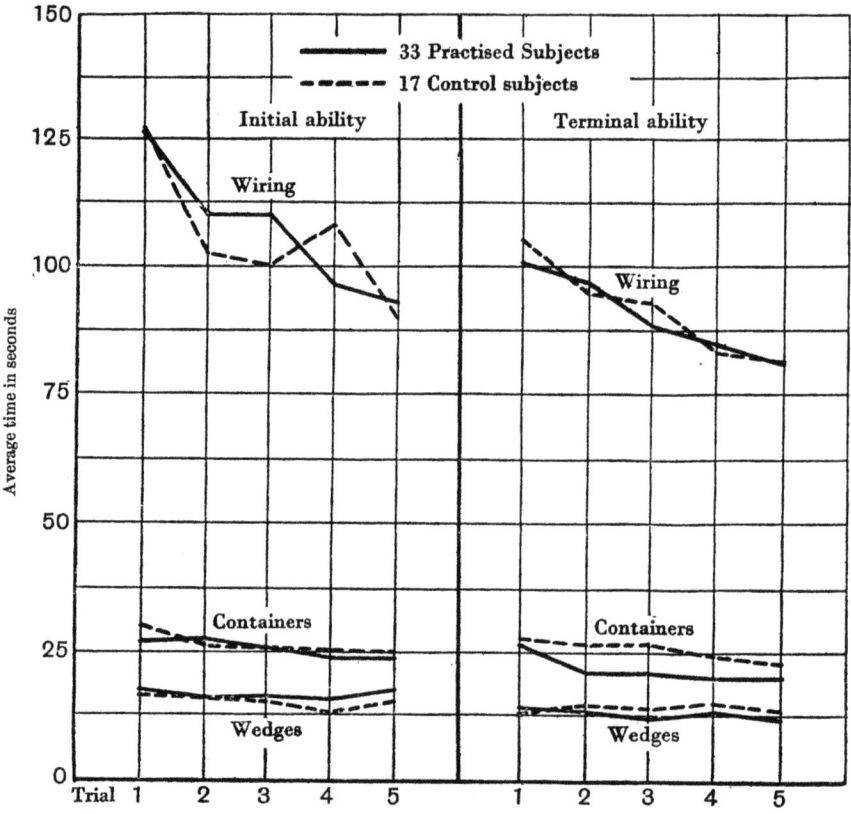

Fig. 26. Comparison between initial and terminal abilities of practised and control groups.

difference is due to initial weakness in the practisers rather than to terminal superiority in the control group, and is too small to attach much significance to. Moreover, it is not verified by the data from the schoolboys.

It is interesting to notice that the terminal measures show, throughout, an improvement over the initial measures, and that little loss in

Table XXXIV.

Schoolboys. Practised groups compared with the control group.

Initial ability

| | Group B | | | | Group A | | | |
	10 screws		10 wedges		5 porcelains		10 containers	
	A	R	A	R	A	R	A	R
Practised groups								
No. of subjects	20	20	20	20	18	16	18	18
Average time (sec.)	43·9	19	167·3	44	406	77·1	141·4	63·4
Probable error	1·18	0·51	3·73	0·87	16·3	3·01	2·95	1·50
Control group								
No. of subjects	32	32	30	30	30	28	28	28
Average time (sec.)	43·4	18·7	153	42·1	400·9	82	159·5	60·3
Probable error	0·73	0·40	3·47	0·79	15·58	1·85	3·88	0·99

Terminal ability

| | Group B | | | | Group A | | | |
	10 screws		10 wedges		5 porcelains		10 containers	
	A	R	A	R	A	R	A	R
Practised groups								
No. of subjects	20	20	20	20	18	16	18	18
Average time (sec.)	40·7	18·2	138	45·4	292·6	69·7	129·5	59·4
Probable error	1·13	0·55	3·03	0·93	10·6	2·86	2·34	1·13
Control group								
No. of subjects	32	32	30	30	30	28	28	28
Average time (sec.)	38·1	17·1	131·5	41·4	355·5	71·5	140·2	55
Probable error	0·58	0·34	3·06	0·78	15·90	1·65	2·42	0·90

Gain

| | Group B | | | | Group A | | | |
	10 screws		10 wedges		5 porcelains		10 containers	
	A	R	A	R	A	R	A	R
Practised groups								
Average time (sec.)	3·2	0·8	29·3	−1·4	113·4	7·4	11·9	4·0
Probable error	0·97	0·41	4·18	0·90	18·1	1·19	2·67	1·63
Control group								
Average time (sec.)	5·3	1·6	21·5	0·7	45·4	10·5	19·3	5·3
Probable error	0·73	0·25	3·16	0·60	18·3	1·68	3·89	1·03

the practice effect seen in the initial measures seems to have occurred during the period which intervened between these and the terminal measures.

C. DATA FROM SCHOOLBOYS

Our schoolboy subjects were divided into two practising groups and a control group. Each of the former practised two double (assembling and stripping) operations. Their practice was, therefore, more extensive and less intensive than that undertaken by the adult groups. Except in the 'screws' operations, their initial and terminal measures were more exhaustive. The measurement for 'wedges' and 'containers' was the average time for five trials, each trial being the assemblage (or stripping) of ten of the objects; for the much longer 'porcelain' operation two trials, of five 'porcelains' each, were given. They were measured at both the 'assembling' and the 'stripping' operations.

The data from these larger groups were treated statistically and are tabulated in Table XXXIV. This gives, for each group, the average time per trial initially and terminally (with their probable errors), the gain shown in the latter over the former, and the probable error of this gain. In only two instances, viz. in 'wedge' assembling and in 'porcelain' assembling, is the improvement shown by the practised subjects greater than that of the controls. Even in these cases the differences are not statistically significant. Thus, in the first instance, the practised subjects improve by 29·3 sec. per trial, the controls by 21·5 sec. and the difference in favour of the practisers is 7·8 sec., with a probable error of 5·2. The difference in the 'porcelain' assembling operation is 68 sec. with a probable error of 25·7. In neither case is the difference sufficiently large in relation to its probable error to justify our attaching much importance to it. We must conclude that nowhere in our data is there any definite evidence of practice at one operation bringing about improvement at another.[1]

---

[1] Reference to the figures and tables of this chapter will show that the practised and control groups were of approximately equal 'initial' ability in most operations. The conclusions of this chapter are confirmed in Chapter XIII, where we are able to compare groups made up by pairing individuals of the same 'initial' ability.

CHAPTER XII

RELATIONS BETWEEN DYNAMIC FUNCTIONS

A. 'ABILITY' AND 'IMPROVABILITY'

In Chapter II, Section B, 'function' was defined as any immediately observable performance as it occurs in its concrete entirety, and 'dynamic' function as one which relates to any change that may occur in the performance. It was also observed in the same chapter that the measurement of a dynamic function may be expressed both as an absolute quantity and as a percentage of that which changes.

Two dynamic functions enter conspicuously into our data, namely, (1) the variation in 'ability' shown from day to day during the practice period, which we shall refer to as 'daily variability', and (2) the improvement in 'ability' brought about by practice, which we shall call 'improvability'. It is the aim of the present chapter to examine the relation of these to one another, and to certain other functions, namely, to 'initial' ability, 'total' ability, and 'intelligence'.

Where we have employed the correlation method, a fair degree of chance fluctuation must be allowed for in the coefficients in view of their large probable errors. These figures are merely intended to express the relations found in the present data in a way that is at once simple and comprehensive. At the same time, where there is general agreement among the several groups (involving altogether eighty practised subjects) and between the different operations practised by the same group, these general indications are not without importance.

1. 'INITIAL' ABILITY COMPARED WITH 'IMPROVABILITY'.

We have already observed a tendency for those of weaker ability initially to make a greater absolute improvement. This fact is clearly indicated in the correlations between 'initial' ability (i.e. on the first day of practice) and absolute 'improvability' given in Table XXXV. In both groups the correlations are negative throughout, and in most cases they are markedly so.

A similar relation holds when we express the improvement as a percentage of the initial ability (Table XXXV), though the figures are

10-2

somewhat smaller and in one case a small positive (but statistically insignificant) correlation occurs.

The general conclusion appears to be that in these routine manual operations an inverse relationship is to be expected between the

Table XXXV.

Correlation of initial ability with (i) absolute improvability, (ii) percentage improvability, and (iii) variability. (Decimal points omitted. A = assembling, B = stripping.)

		Screws		Wedges		Porcelains		Containers	
		A	S	A	S	A	S	A	S
Absolute improvability	Adults	−83	−79	−76	−61	−89	−45	−90	−69
	Schoolboys	−75	−80	−66	−79	−47	−70	−31	−38
Percentage improvability	Adults	−60	−38	−65	−43	−32	23	−83	−09
	Schoolboys	−66	−59	−67	−73	−35	−51	−14	−34
Variability	Adults	−52	−52	−22	24	−88	−38	−73	·05
	Schoolboys	−55	01	02	09	−58	−23	−43	−26

ability shown at first and the absolute amount of improvement that follows from subsequent practice, and that when the improvement is expressed as a percentage of the initial ability the inverse nature of the relationship becomes less marked.

2. TOTAL 'ABILITY' COMPARED WITH 'IMPROVABILITY'.

Closely similar results are obtained when we compare 'improvability' with the total ability shown over the whole practice period. To indicate where departures from the general rule occur we have represented these data graphically. Some of these graphs are shown in figs. 27–32.[1] The relation of total ability to absolute improvability is shown by a continuous line, and its relation to percentage improvability by a broken line. In comparing the curves for adults with those for schoolboys it must be remembered that the latter had considerably less practice at each operation. Occasionally the boys' curve passes below the abscissa. This does not mean that the individual in question actually got worse during practice, but that he happened to do worse on the last day—our measure of 'improvability' being the excess of the time taken on the first day over that taken on the last. It will usually follow, of course, that he has made little real progress.

[1] See footnote to p. 49.

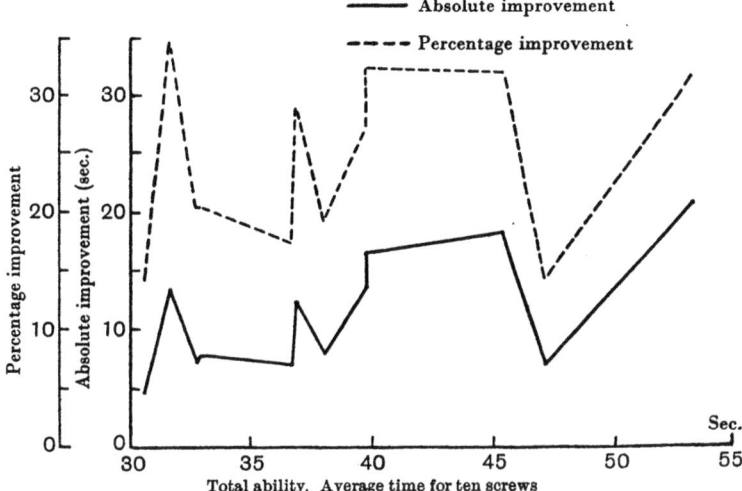

Fig. 27. Total ability compared with absolute and percentage improvability at assembling screws. Twelve adults.

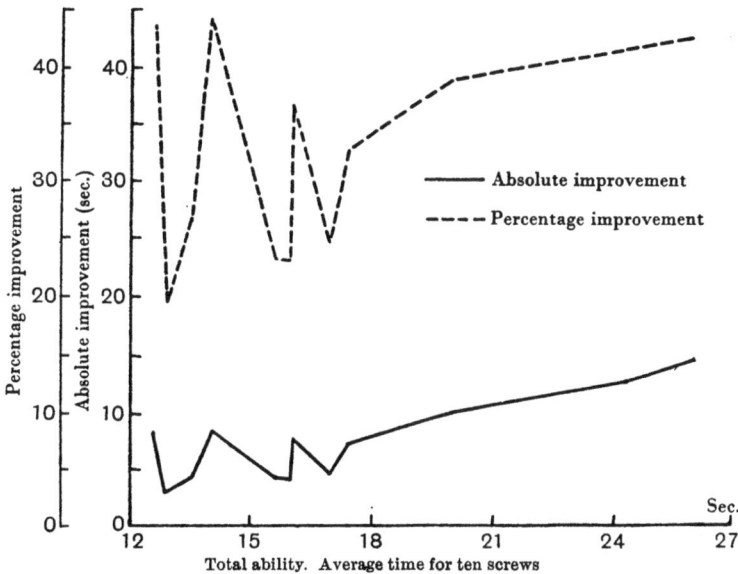

Fig. 28. Total ability compared with absolute and percentage improvability at stripping screws. Twelve adults.

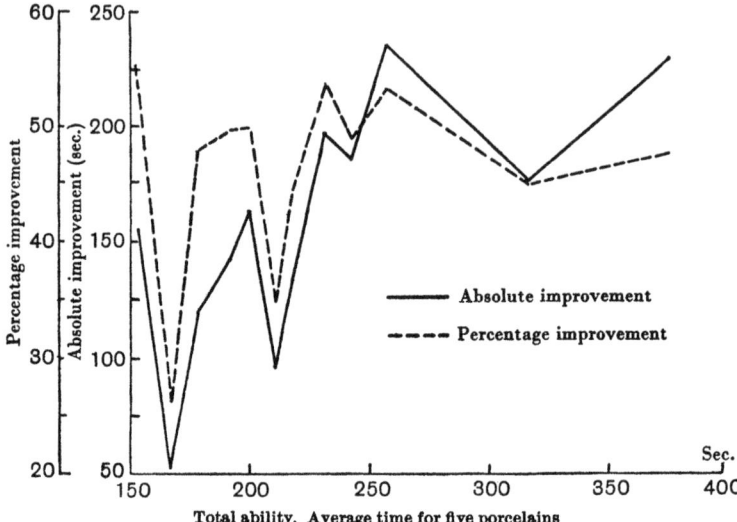

Fig. 29. Total ability compared with absolute and percentage improvability at assembling porcelains. Twelve adults.

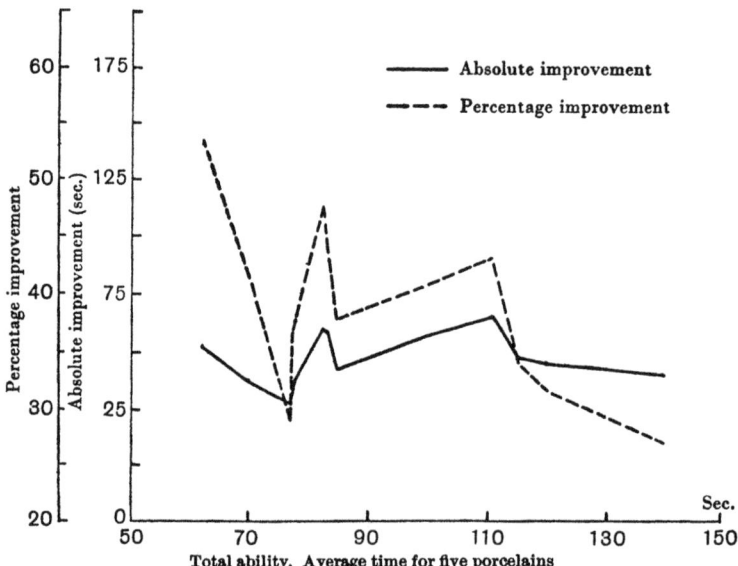

Fig. 30. Total ability compared with absolute and percentage improvability at stripping porcelains. Twelve adults.

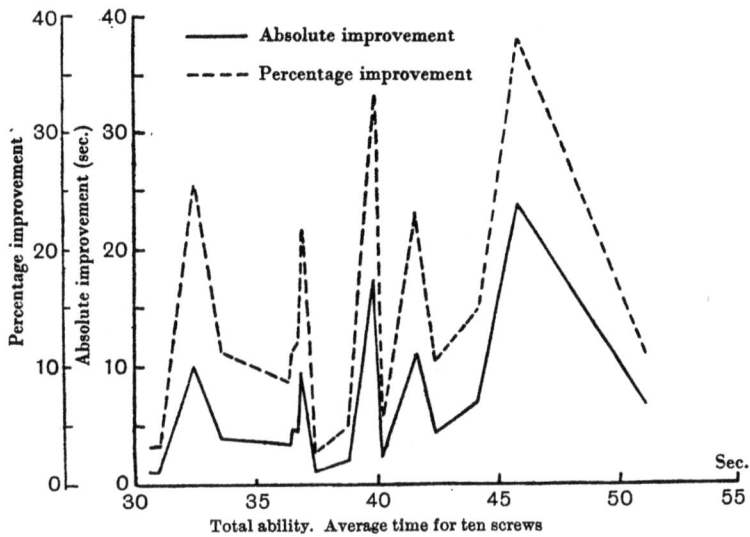

Fig. 31. Total ability compared with absolute and percentage improvability at assembling screws. Eighteen boys.

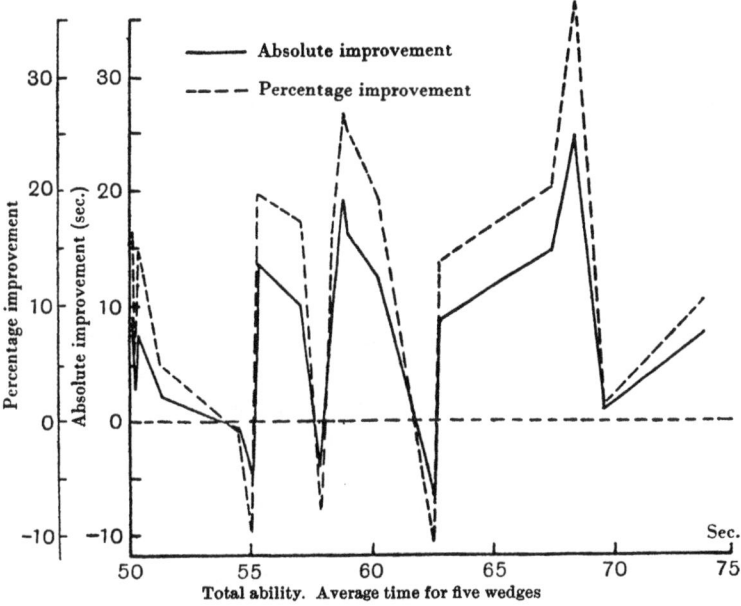

Fig. 32. Total ability compared with absolute and percentage improvability at assembling wedges. Nineteen boys.

A general rise in the curve from left to right indicates an inverse relationship between total ability and the improvability (absolute or percentage) with which it is compared. Such is clearly seen in all the curves for assembling and stripping screws (cf. figs. 27, 28 and 31) and in the adult curve for assembling porcelains (fig. 29). The same general tendency is also evident in the boys' curves for stripping wedges and for assembling and stripping porcelains and in the adult curves for assembling and stripping containers, although, in these latter, large individual departures from the general rule are to be seen.

Of the remaining curves, the adult curve for stripping wedges shows a tendency to greater improvability at both ends of the scale of total ability, and the remainder take a more or less jagged horizontal course indicating little relationship, either positive or negative, between the items compared (cf. figs. 30 and 32). Nowhere do we find indications of a positive correlation.

On the whole, the curves suggest that total ability tends to be related to improvability in much the same way as is initial ability, except that the inverse relation is less marked.[1]

3. RATE OF PROGRESS AT THE SAME LEVEL OF ABILITY.

So far we have been concerned with the total improvement shown over the whole period of practice. We have now to consider the rate of progress at a given point on the scale of 'ability'. We have already noticed a tendency for initial progress and for the average progress made over the whole period to be greater in those subjects who rank lower on the scale. Both initial rate and average rate are necessarily measured over that part of the scale to which the subject attains, and the superior rate of slower subjects may well be due to progress being more readily made (when measured in the same units) at lower levels of ability—just as an individual makes more rapid progress at first. We shall now inquire how far this may indeed be the case. Will the superior rate be maintained after the weaker subject has caught up to the point on the scale of ability at which the faster subject started?

---

[1] The negative correlations found with these manual operations are in contrast with the high positive correlations found by Flügel between ability and absolute improvability in mental operations (adding numbers). See J. C. Flügel, *Practice, Fatigue and Oscillation* (*Brit. Journ. Psychol.*, Monograph Suppt. No. 13, 1928). A similar, though lower, positive relation was found by Wimms for the same operation (addition), which tended, however, to diminish to zero in the case of more complex operations (multiplying four digits). See J. H. Wimms, "The relative effects of fatigue and practice produced by different kinds of mental work" (*Brit. Journ. Psychol.* 1907, ii, No. 2, pp. 153–95).

How will their rates compare when both are travelling over the same part of the scale?

Seeing that some of the practice curves cross, while others, on reaching the same point on the scale, do not, it is clear that all will not conform to the same law. As before, we shall be concerned with general tendencies rather than with hard and fast rules. The discovery of general tendencies is of obvious practical value when dealing with large numbers, and may shed light on important theoretical questions. In the present instance the general relation which may be found between ability and rate of progress has an important bearing on the theory of learning.

In order to see more clearly the general courses of progress, we have first smoothed the practice curves by averaging each point on the curve with the point on either side of it. Thus, the first point on the curve represents the average performance over the first, second and third days; the second point is the average of the second, third and fourth days, and so on. These smoothed curves are shown in figs. 10 and 11.[1]

Two horizontal lines were then drawn on each chart at such positions that they would cut the majority of the curves and so mark off a range on the scale of ability common to this majority. These are the lines BX, CY in each figure. The part of the chart lying between these lines was drawn to a larger scale to show more clearly the slopes of the curves in this region. Finally, to compare more easily their slopes, the curves were transferred laterally so as to begin at a common point. These are shown in figs. 33–37.[2] They afford a ready means of comparing the rate at which individuals of different ability progressed over the same part of the scale.

On examining these latter figures it is at once evident that certain individual curves depart widely from their fellows. This occurs where the individual is reaching the limits of his 'improvability', or is approaching, or emerging from, a 'plateau'. Such are seen in the curves of O, Gr (fig. 33), Gra, Or (fig. 34), M, Wal (fig. 35), P, M (fig. 36). We have already seen that the occurrence of plateaux, and the point at which the so-called limits of practice are reached, are individual characteristics. These parts of the curve, as also the initial stages of practice, will hardly be expected to conform in slope to any

[1] For 'screws' and 'porcelains' only; see footnote to p. 49.

[2] See the above footnote. Precisely similar results were found in the data from 'containers' and 'wedges'.

general rule that may be found to underlie the slope of the more normal part of the curve. They, together with similar instances that appear in

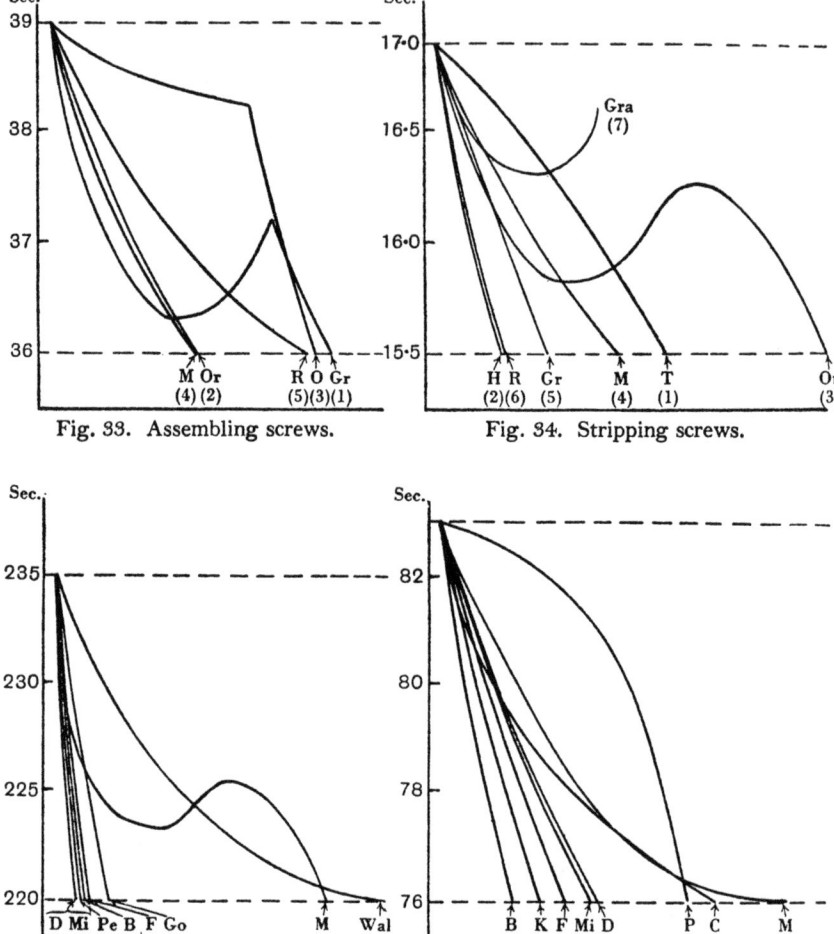

Fig. 33. Assembling screws.

Fig. 34. Stripping screws.

Fig. 35. Assembling porcelains.

Fig. 36. Stripping porcelains.

Figs. 33–36. Rate at which persons of different ability progress over the same part of the scale. The numbers in brackets denote order of merit on the first day of practice.

the other figures, may, therefore, be dismissed as easily explicable departures from the more normal course of progress seen in the other curves *at the level of ability under examination.* It is in the more normal curves, where progress is unmistakable and more or less uniform, that a possible connection between 'ability' and 'rate of progress' must be sought.

On examining these curves, it will, however, be seen that there are still individual differences in rate of progress, notwithstanding the common range of ability over which it is now being measured, for the curves are not even approximately coincident. We must, therefore, conclude that the rate of progress will still tend to vary from one individual to another as the same range of 'ability' is traversed, even where the above-mentioned special phases of the practice curve are not involved. Nevertheless, many striking instances are seen where individuals of widely different 'ability' progress at the same rate while passing over the same part of the scale; as witness the curves of H and R (fig. 34), of D and Pe (fig. 35), and of D and Mi (fig. 36).

Many of the curves of our slower subjects do not fall within the range of ability so far examined. We have, accordingly, made a further comparison of these at the lower point on the scale necessitated by their position on the chart. These are shown in fig. 37. They again indicate individual differences and provide even more striking evidence that persons widely apart on the scale of 'ability' may progress at the same rate while passing over the same part of the scale.

We may now attempt to answer the main question which led to this analysis—how are these individual differences in rate of progress at the same level of ability related to the ability displayed by the individual on the first day of practice? A comparison of the curves[1] fails to disclose any definite relationship, either positive or negative, between these two functions. Sometimes the more able subject makes the greater progress over this particular part of the scale, sometimes the less able. The same result ensues on comparing rate with ability as judged by the length of practice needed to attain to the point on the scale at which the rate is measured. Our general conclusion must be that neither a person's initial performance nor the length of practice he requires to attain to a given level of ability affords any criterion for judging the rate at which he may progress beyond that level under the same conditions of practice.

To sum up the results of this section, it may be said, briefly, that under similar conditions of practice the weaker subjects will tend to make greater progress than, but not to surpass, those of superior

[1] Figs. 33–37, and similarly as regards the 'containers' and 'wedges' operations.

ability, as judged either by initial performance or by their total output over the practice period; but the chances are even as to which will progress at the greater pace while traversing the same part of the scale of ability.

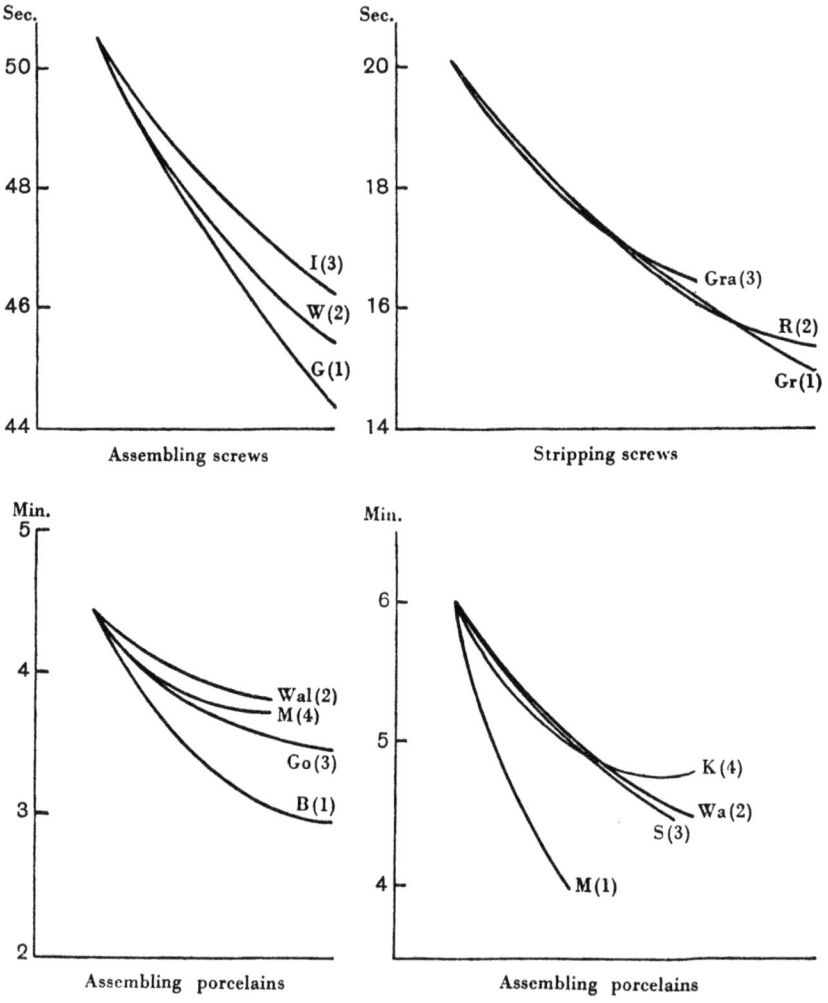

Fig. 37. Rate at which persons of different ability progress over the same part of the scale. The numbers in brackets denote order of merit on the first day of practice.

B. 'ABILITY' AND 'VARIABILITY'

1. 'INITIAL' ABILITY COMPARED WITH 'VARIABILITY'.

Table XXXV gives the correlations between initial ability and daily variability. Nowhere is there any appreciable positive correlation and in many cases a high inverse relationship is indicated. These coefficients thus afford verification of, and numerical expression to, the fact already suggested in the individual curves, that on the whole the initially weaker subjects tend to exhibit greater daily variability. The figures suggest that this relationship is more marked in assembling than in stripping—especially where the more complex 'porcelain' and 'container' material is concerned.

2. 'TOTAL' ABILITY COMPARED WITH 'VARIABILITY'.

The comparison of daily variability with total ability (over the practice period) is shown graphically in figs. 38–40. As before, a general rise in the curve from left to right indicates an inverse relationship. Such occurs in many of these curves, and nowhere is there evidence of positive correlation. The inverse relationship is most clearly seen in those operations where there exists a high negative correlation (over 0·5) between initial ability and variability (cf. Table XXXV). This is in accordance with the already noted tendency for initial ability to correlate with total ability. On the whole, it appears more marked in the right-hand end of the curves, i.e. in the weaker subjects. Examples of this type of curve are shown in fig. 38.

In the remaining operations the general horizontal course of the curve suggests the absence of any marked relationship—either positive or negative. Examples are shown in fig. 39. In certain instances, as shown in fig. 40, an initial fall in the curve suggests a positive correlation in this particular part of the scale, but the numbers involved here are too few to throw much light on general tendencies.

C. 'IMPROVABILITY' AND 'VARIABILITY'

Table XXXVI gives the correlations between daily variability and improvability measured (i) in the absolute sense, and (ii) as a percentage of initial ability. Where the correlations are of any appreciable magnitude (over 0·4), they are, with one exception (stripping wedges), positive. This conforms with our previous findings, for if, as we have

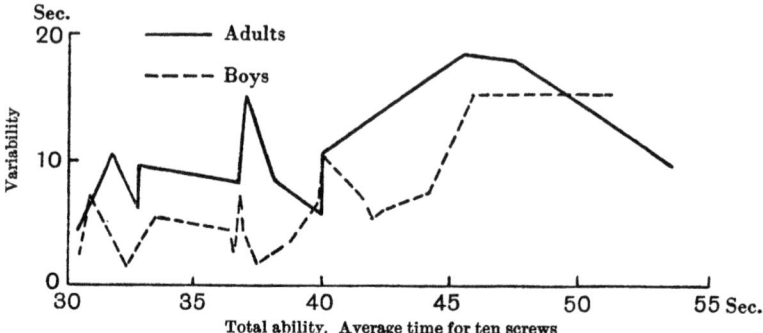

Fig. 38. Total ability compared with daily variability at assembling screws.

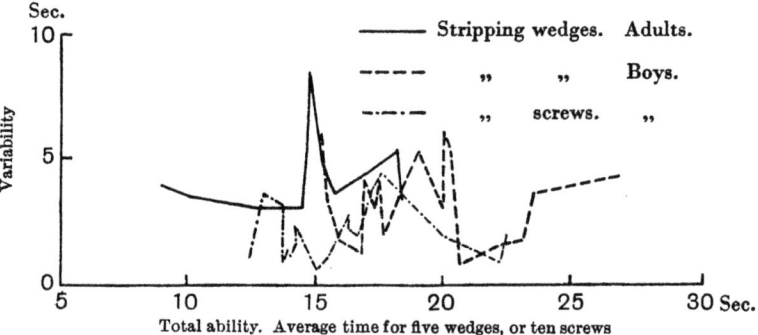

Fig. 39. Total ability compared with variability.

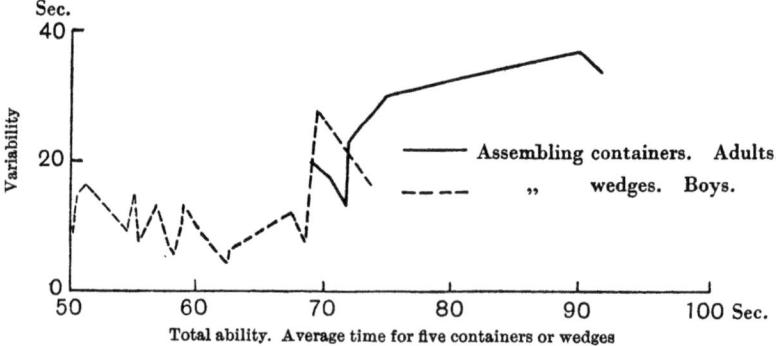

Fig. 40. Total ability compared with variability.

seen, those who are at first most able improve least and vary least, it is understandable that those who improve least should also vary least.

Table XXXVI.

Correlation of variability with (i) absolute improvability, and (ii) percentage improvability. (Decimal points omitted. A = assembling, B = stripping.)

		Screws		Wedges		Porcelains		Containers	
		A	S	A	S	A	S	A	S
Absolute	Adults	43	43	22	−69	58	−35	73	−01
improvability	Schoolboys	37	−13	−06	−29	−05	22	−26	47
Percentage	Adults	19	04	00	−56	41	00	62	−07
improvability	Schoolboys	34	−17	−11	−28	−08	40	−28	47

In other cases, the relation tends to zero rather than to any marked negative correlation.[1] On the whole, the positive correlation between improvability and variability appears lower than the negative correlation which each of these show with initial ability (Table XXXV).

D. 'IMPROVABILITY' AND 'INTELLIGENCE'

We may inquire, finally, how far general intelligence, as measured by the intelligence test, is an indication of ability to improve by practice at these routine operations. The practical importance of such knowledge in the work of vocational guidance and selection is too obvious to need comment. It has also great theoretical interest as shedding light on the nature of the influences affecting improvability.

The relevant correlations are given in Table XXXVII. Unfortunately some of our practised adult subjects were unable to take the intelligence test, and this reduced the number available for the data of the table for 'screws', 'wedges', 'porcelains' and 'containers', to eight, eleven, ten and six respectively. In these circumstances, the figures must not, of course, be taken at their face value. They are intended merely to indicate whether, in the present data, there was a tendency for those who did better at the intelligence test to improve more by practice at the routine operations. Such a relation is seen in the figures for the porcelain operations, in both 'assembling' and 'stripping', and for both measures of 'improvability'. But the same

[1] With the exception of the adult figures for stripping wedges—but the subjects are too few to permit of a conclusion from this group alone.

high figures are not found for the other operations, although those for 'assembling' are in every case but one (− 0·10) positive. So far as they go, they suggest that 'intelligence' may have played a larger part in determining progress at the more complex operations.

Table XXXVII.

Correlation of 'intelligence' with (i) absolute improvability, and (ii) percentage improvability. (Decimal points omitted. A = assembling, S = stripping.)

		Screws		Wedges		Porcelains		Containers	
		A	S	A	S	A	S	A	S
Absolute	Adults	30	−05	10	−10	62	79	17	−69
improvability	Schoolboys	−45	−35	−54	−40	17	−47	34	16
Percentage	Adults	43	76	−10	−22	54	51	72	−66
improvability	Schoolboys	−45	−31	−54	−32	19	−34	37	09

A similar suggestion emerges from the figures for the larger boys' groups, where the correlations for the more complex operations of assembling porcelains and containers, although not large enough to indicate a significant positive relation, are at least higher than the negative correlations seen in the other operations.

More commonly, however, there is to be seen in these tables—and especially so in the boys—an inverse relation between ability at the 'intelligence' test and the improvement (both 'absolute' and 'percentage') made at the operations. This is readily understandable when it is remembered that the amount of improvement depends, in part, on the subject's ability at first. We have seen that initial ability was related inversely to 'improvability', but directly to 'intelligence'. It is, therefore, not unreasonable to find a tendency to inverse relationship between 'improvability' and 'intelligence'.

This does not mean that the possession of intelligence is a handicap to progress at these operations. Comparison of these tables with the correlations between improvability and initial ability (Table XXXV) shows the inverse relation to be higher throughout in the latter. The suggestion is that superior intelligence is an asset to progress, but that this advantage is more than offset by the superior initial ability which accompanies superior intelligence and which makes further progress more difficult (as shown by its inverse correlation with improvability).

Improvability must depend on several factors, among which are the ability with which the person starts and his intelligence. The analysis of these factors must not be confused with the simple comparisons provided in the present data. The most these can do is to show how unsafe it would be to draw inferences about an individual's capacity to improve at these routine operations merely on the basis of his general intelligence, and without considering the proficiency to which he has already attained. Furthermore, when all three functions (ability, improvability and intelligence) are considered together, our data nowhere support the view that the good 'brain-worker' is necessarily a poor 'manual' worker.

E. SUMMARY

The general indications of the data examined in the present chapter may be briefly summarized as follows:

There is a general and, in some cases, a high inverse relationship between 'initial' ability and 'improvability' (both 'absolute' and 'percentage') at the routine assembling operations. A similar, though less marked, relationship appears to hold between 'total' ability and these measures of improvability.

A like tendency towards inverse relationship is frequently seen between 'daily variability' and 'ability' (both 'initial' and 'total'). It appears somewhat higher where 'initial' ability and the more complex operations are concerned.

The relation of 'improvability' to 'variability' is less uniform. Where the correlations are highest, they are, with one exception, positive. Negative correlations also appear in some operations, but, apart from the exception noted, they are too small to be important.

'Improvability' (both 'absolute' and 'percentage') tends to an inverse relationship with 'intelligence'. Comparison of these functions with 'initial' ability suggests that this is due to the handicap to further progress imposed by an accompanying greater initial ability, rather than to any hindrance arising out of a superior intelligence. It appears probable from the tables that where 'ability' is equal initially, the greater improvement would fall to those who do better at the intelligence test.

CHAPTER XIII

THE TRANSFER OF 'TRAINING'
EFFECTS

A. SOME FURTHER QUESTIONS

1. 'PRACTICE' DISTINGUISHED FROM 'TRAINING'.

It will be remembered that the subjects who practised the assembling operations, and so provided the data examined in Chapter XI, did so by repeating the operation at maximum speed for a given number of times. They were given no instructions on the manner in which the operation might best be carried out, but were left entirely to their own devices in that matter. In accordance with our usage of the term throughout, we shall continue to call such uninstructed and more or less mechanical repetition, 'practice'.

When it became evident from the data examined in Chapter XI that the effects of this kind of practice seldom 'transfer', it became important to inquire how far this negative result might be due to the nature of the practice. In order to determine this, a further experiment, to be described in the present chapter, was carried out. Here our subjects were instructed in the general principles underlying the best methods of work, and they carried out formal exercises designed to direct attention to points to be observed in manipulating the material. To distinguish this method from the above-described 'practice', we shall refer to it as 'training'.[1]

2. How does the effect transfer?

There are two conceivable ways in which the effects of practice or of training may transfer; the transference may result in an increase in 'ability', or as an increase in 'improvability', or, of course, as both. In the former case, the transferred effect will be manifested by an immediate increase in ability at the operation subsequently undertaken;

[1] A similar distinction between 'practice' and 'training' has been previously made by Dr C. S. Myers who, in a paper on 'Educability' addressed to the British Association in 1928, wrote: "A fundamental distinction must be drawn between (a) the mechanical repetitive practice of an innate ability...and (b) that higher training which leads to the acquisition of the best attitude, the best technique and style and an adequate knowledge of general guiding principles enabling the best use to be made of an innate ability".

in the latter case, it will be shown by an increased rate of progress as practice at the subsequent operation continues. In Chapter XI our examination of the transfer question was necessarily confined to the sphere of 'ability'. The data which we have now to examine will permit an extension of this inquiry into the region of 'improvability'.

3. THE MEASUREMENT OF IMPROVEMENT.

Experiments in transfer involve the measurement and comparison of the improvement shown by different individuals (practisers and controls) at some given operation. Our examination of the practice curves has indicated that progress is by no means uniform, but tends to diminish as efficiency increases. In conformity therewith, individuals ranking low on the scale of ability were found to make greater improvement for a given amount of practice than those who stood initially higher, and this was true whether the improvement were measured in absolute units or as a percentage of the ability with which the individual started. It follows that any estimate of the effect of practice, or of training, must take account of the position on the scale of ability at which the effect is produced. The effect is not necessarily greater in an individual whose score (in speed) is improved from 100 to 80 sec. than in one whose score is raised from 40 to 30 sec. Only between persons of equal 'initial' or 'terminal' ability are such comparisons safely made.

B. FURTHER EVIDENCE RELATING TO 'PRACTICE'

The operation in which our subjects were 'trained' in the experiment to be described later was that of assembling containers. Consequently, it was desirable to make a more detailed study of the effects of 'practice' at this operation than was possible with the limited adult group examined in Chapter XI, in order that a closer comparison with the effects of 'training' in relation to the above questions might be possible. The number of adult practisers at containers was, therefore, increased to thirteen and the number of controls to thirty-one, the same plan and procedure being followed as before. From these were drawn groups of equal 'initial' ability by the pairing of as many practised individuals as possible with controls making the same initial score.[1] These groups were strictly comparable, both as regards their total

---

[1] Within a degree well within the limits of experimental error.

(or average) initial scores and the initial scores of the individuals composing them. The scores included within each group covered a wide range of individual ability.

The initial and terminal scores of these groups are given in figs. 41 and 42, where the five points of the graph indicate, as before, the times taken to execute the five successive trials which constituted the test.[1] The 'terminal' graphs in these figures confirm our previous observations, since nowhere do they indicate a superiority of the practised subjects over the controls.[2]

Table XXXVIII.

Showing difference between mean gain of 'practisers' and that of initially equal 'controls', with standard error of the difference (sec.).

Test	Practisers	Controls	Difference	Standard error
Assembling screws	23·3	22·7	+ 0·6	16·5
Stripping screws	8·6	9·5	− 0·9	5·7
Porcelains	50·4	86·3	−35·9	31·6
Wedges	6·4	12·4	− 6·0	10·3
Wiring	73·9	30·1	+43·8	38·3

The same data are shown statistically in Table XXXVIII. This gives, for each operation, (*a*) the average improvement made by the practised group (i.e. the mean value in seconds of the initial score minus the terminal score), (*b*) that made by the controls of equal initial ability, (*c*) the difference, and (*d*) the standard error of the difference. Only in the case of wiring is there a difference of any magnitude in favour of the practisers, and this barely exceeds its standard error.

C. THE 'TRAINING' EXPERIMENT

1. GENERAL PLAN.

We have further to consider the 'training' experiment. This was carried out after the data discussed in Chapter XI had been examined. The same general plan and conditions were adhered to as in these

---

[1] With the exception of 'wedges' which are here shown by a single point giving the total of the five trials, since the trials were not timed separately.
[2] The apparent superiority in the first three terminal trials at wiring is not statistically significant. See Table XXXVIII.

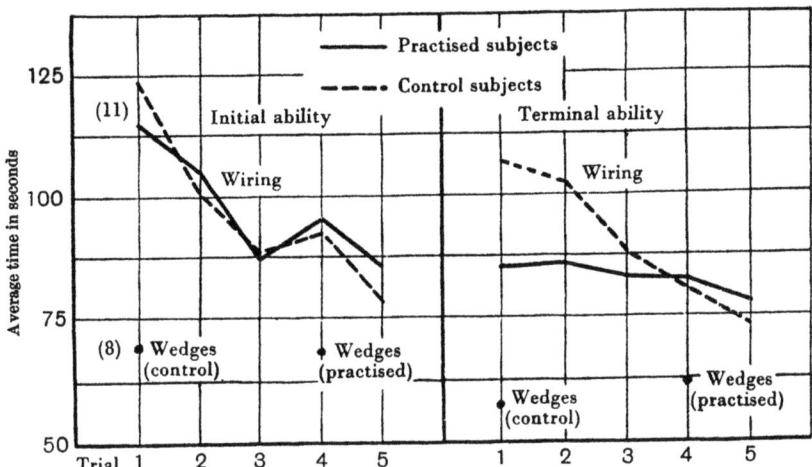

Fig. 41. Comparison between terminal ability of practised and of control groups of equal initial ability. (Number of subjects in brackets.)

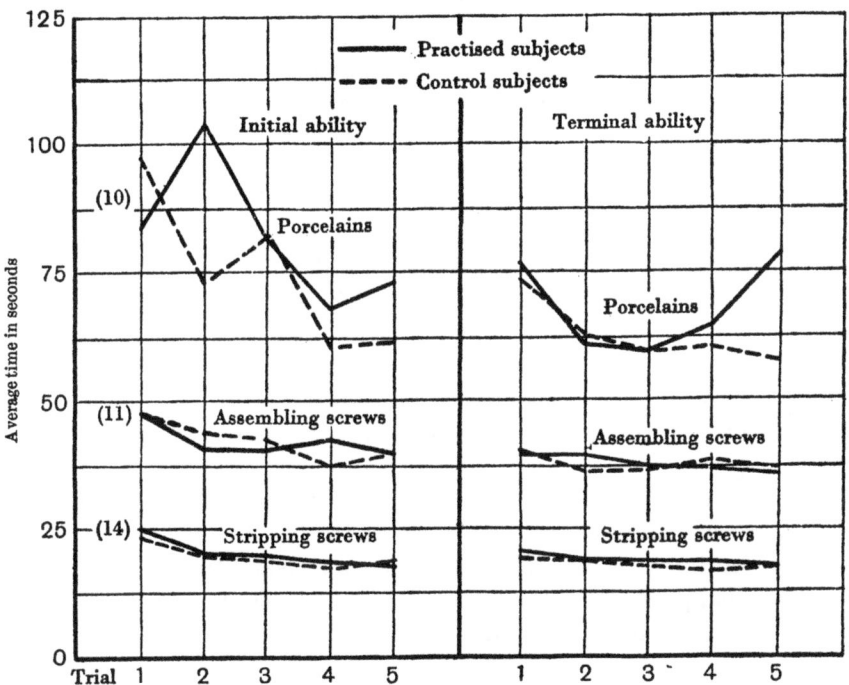

Fig. 42. Comparison between terminal ability of practised and of control groups of equal initial ability. (Number of subjects in brackets.)

former 'practice' experiments, with the exception that the high-speed repetitive practice, which intervened between the initial tests and the terminal re-tests, was now replaced by training, in which the subject effected far fewer repetitions of the operation but, in the time thus saved, was given instruction in general principles and specific points relating to the best methods of carrying out the assembling operation. Thirty-six new subjects, similar in character to our former adults, were tested as before, 'trained' on the container operation, and then re-tested. The eleven daily training periods were of approximately the same length as the former practice periods; and the initial and terminal testing took the same form as in the practice experiment.

2. THE TRAINING SCHEME.

The 'training' was based upon an introspective analysis of the mental activities involved in carrying out these manual operations (which the writer had practised), and on observations made while watching the previous subjects at 'practice'. The aim of the course was to impart a knowledge of certain general principles underlying the skilful handling of assembly material and to provide specific exercise in applying them to *one* assembling operation, viz. the container operation. The scheme fell into two sections; in Section I the general principles were explained, while Section II consisted of special exercises, based on the container operation, which the trainee was asked to carry out. These exercises aimed at showing how to apply the principles. They fell into five groups as follows.

The first group of exercises dealt with such matters of 'general method' as the arrangement of parts on the bench,[1] their order of assembly and the manner of holding them.

The second group may be called 'eye observation exercises': they showed what to observe through the eyes, while engaged on the assembly operation.

The third group may be called, correspondingly, 'finger observation exercises': they indicated the things to be observed through the fingers. In the eye exercises, the trainee was asked to *look* carefully at what was happening and to pay special regard to certain visual aspects of the shapes of the items and to the spatial relationship into which

---

[1] The matter of arrangement was included here for completeness but was not allowed to enter as a factor in the 'terminal' tests. These were performed under the same external conditions as applied to the 'initial' tests.

they should be brought. In the finger exercises, he was required to pay special attention to the 'feelings' in his *fingers* as they carried out the movements and to notice carefully certain aspects of this experience. Just exactly what to notice was made clear in each exercise.

The fourth group comprised exercises in the 'control of attention and of effort': they aimed at showing how these may be most economically employed throughout the operation.

The fifth and last group afforded practice in applying the results of the foregoing exercises to the operation as a whole under normal conditions of work.

This scheme was carried out in the form of eleven 'lessons' corresponding in time to the periods devoted to 'practice' by our previous groups. Each lesson opened with a brief (verbal) revision of the chief points already dealt with. Attention was then directed to the 'point' of the next exercise, which was explained and demonstrated by the trainer. The subjects did the exercises themselves, paying special attention to the point in question. Each exercise was repeated several times, the whole being treated as an observation exercise rather than one of mere speed. When all the exercises had been taken (by the eighth or ninth day according to the group), the remaining days were devoted to revising the chief points, and to dealing with points (bad methods, etc.) observed in individuals during the speed tests with which each lesson concluded and which constituted the subject's daily measure of ability.

The speed tests consisted in first 'assembling' and then 'stripping' five containers, and were worked as follows: days 1 to 7, once; days 8 and 9, twice; days 10 and 11, three times.

Thus, altogether, the 'training' consisted of talks, exercises based on the container operation, and eighty-five repetitions of this operation, as compared with the 440 repetitions which constituted the 'practice' of our former subjects.

3. RESULTS.

(a) *The effect on 'ability'.* As the data were obtained, they were examined graphically as before. After the training, each of the trained groups showed a marked superiority over the 'controls' in the various operations for which they were tested (tests of 'terminal' ability). These differences were so large as to suggest at once that the effect of the 'training' had transferred to the other operations. The issue was, however, complicated by the fact that some difference in ability was observable between the controls and the trained groups before the training was given (i.e. in the 'initial' scores). To overcome this difficulty, as before (cf. p. 163) we paired, with respect to each operation, as many trained individuals as possible with partners of equal initial ability selected from among the controls. Thus were obtained groups which were strictly comparable both as regards total and individual scores. The resulting graphs are given in figs. 43 and 44, where it is seen that in every case the trained subjects are much superior to the controls with whom they formerly scored equally.

Table XXXIX.

Mean gain of 'trainees' and that of initially equal 'controls', with standard error of difference (seconds).

Test	Trainees	Controls	Difference	Standard error
Assembling screws	36·9	11·0	+ 25·9	7·11
Stripping screws	33·8	8·7	+ 25·1	3·75
Porcelains	163·0	63·3	+ 99·7	27·96
Wedges	20·6	4·7	+ 15·9	6·12
Wiring	161·6	56·3	+105·3	32·4

Since the terminal superiority, as shown in the graphs, is an average result, it remained to determine its statistical significance. This was done by computing how far the average terminal improvement shown by the trainees exceeded that of the controls, and the standard error of this difference. The results are given in Table XXXIX. In every operation except wedges, the difference well exceeds three times its standard error; and in the wedges operation it closely approaches this standard. The terminal superiority of the trainees must, therefore, be considered as statistically significant.

(b) *The effect on 'improvability'*. So far, our study of training has been confined to an examination of its effect on the ability shown in the terminal tests. We may now consider its effect on improvability— how far does 'training' influence one's *rate of progress* at an operation subsequently practised? For this purpose, thirty-five of our trained subjects practised the wedges operation under the same conditions as held for our former practisers (i.e. the untrained group). As the data were obtained, the results were plotted in the form of graphs shown in fig. 45. These show the average time taken to assemble five wedges

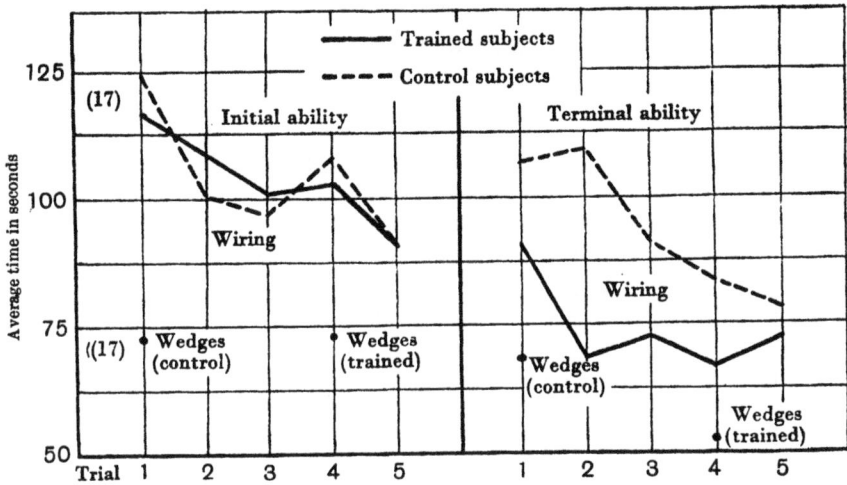

Fig. 43. Comparison between terminal ability of trained and control groups of equal initial ability. (Number of subjects in brackets.)

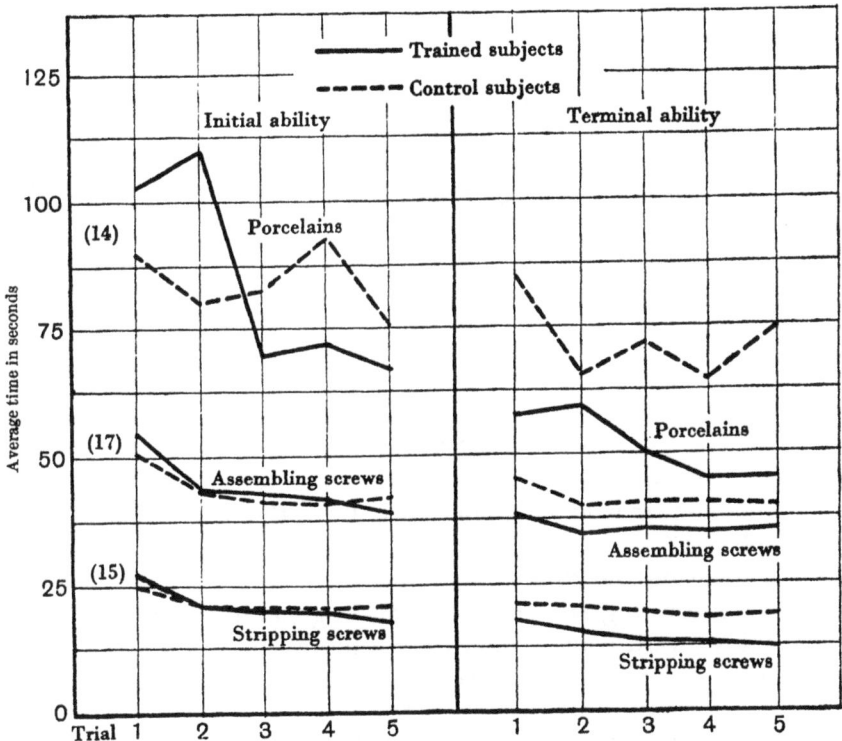

Fig. 44. Comparison between terminal ability of trained and control groups of equal initial ability. (Number of subjects in brackets.)

(one 'trial') over each successive half-practice (twenty-five wedges) by (*a*) three groups of subjects previously trained on containers and (*b*) two groups of untrained subjects. The graphs showing the results of combining the (*a*) groups and the (*b*) groups are indicated by deeper continuous and broken lines respectively. The untrained subjects number eleven throughout; of the trained subjects, thirty-five completed

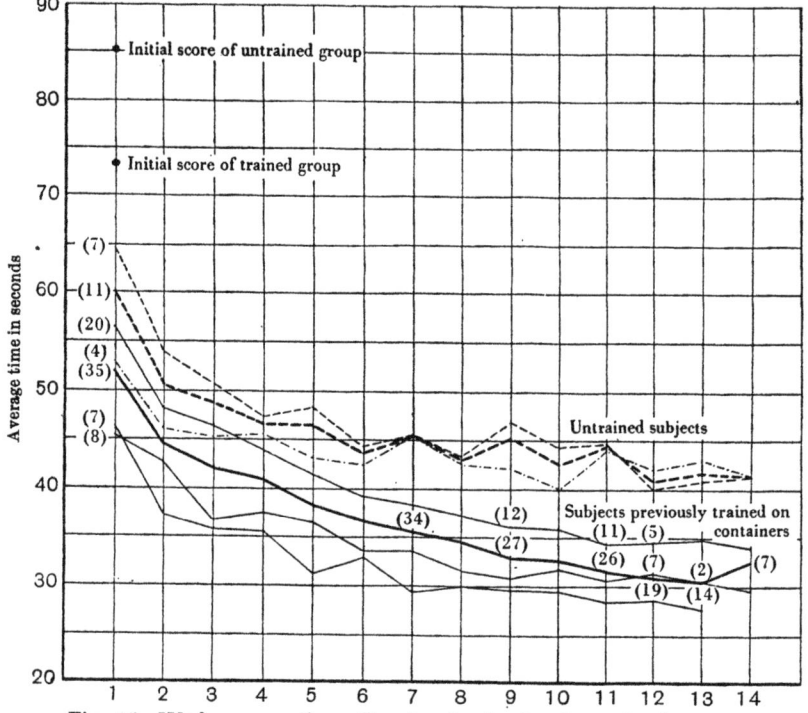

Fig. 45. Wedges operation. Graphs of trained and untrained groups.
(Number of subjects in brackets.)

the first three days' practice (the first six points on the graph), after which the number who were able to continue the practice is given on the graph itself.

On comparing the graphs of trained with those of untrained subjects, the interesting fact emerges that, in general, the former take a steeper downward course, indicating a more rapid rate of progress, than do the latter.[1] Whereas we have invariably found curves of un-

[1] The difference for the whole task (twenty-five wedges) at any point of practice is, of course, five times as large as the difference shown between curves in the figure, since the curves indicate the times taken to do one-fifth of this work.

trained subjects to draw closer together as practice continues (as do their curves in fig. 45), it will be seen that the curves of the trained subjects tend to draw farther away from those of the untrained subjects, owing to their more rapid descent. This means that not only is the rate of progress of the trained subjects greater than that of the untrained subjects actually represented in the figures, but much more so than we should have reason to expect of untrained subjects who had attained to the speeds actually achieved at any point by the trained subjects.

While fig. 45 has enabled us to compare usefully all the data with respect to *relative rates* of improvement, it would be erroneous to suppose that the *absolute differences* in ability, shown between the trained and the untrained groups as practice proceeds, are wholly attributable to the training factor, because these groups were not of equal ability at the beginning.[1] Valid comparisons of this kind are possible only between groups initially equal in ability. We have, therefore, paired off as many as possible of our trained subjects with untrained subjects of equal initial ability at the wedges operation (as measured by the wedges test which immediately preceded the practice at wedges). The practice curves of these initially equal groups, thus selected from the data of fig. 45, are shown in fig. 46: whence it is evident that the group which enjoyed the previous training excels over the untrained group from the first day of practice and maintains a higher rate of progress afterwards.[2]

Although the result just mentioned is based upon the limited number who could be thus paired as equal, it is not unprofitable to ask how far this observed difference between the two groups is statistically significant, for, only in the light of such statistical check can it be seen whether the difference is typical of the groups as a whole or whether, on the contrary, it arises from the abnormal performances of one or two individuals. We have therefore determined the standard error of the difference between the gains (in time score) made by the groups over the first four days of practice (i.e. up to points 7 and 8 of the graphs). This proves to be 1·93 sec. Seeing that the difference itself (9·9 sec.) exceeds five times this value, it can hardly have arisen from the chance variations of individual scores. It seems most readily explained by the training (on containers) which the superior group had received before

[1] And similarly as regards the absolute improvement made by the groups.
[2] As before, the absolute time differences between the groups for the whole task (twenty-five 'wedges') is five times greater than the difference shown by the graphs (five 'wedges').

beginning this period of practice. The effect of such training seems clearly to have transferred in both a 'static' and a 'dynamic' sense, for not only are the trained subjects of superior ability at any given point of the curve, but their potentiality for further improvement under similar conditions of practice is greater.

(*c*) *Comparison between practice and training curves.* Finally, we may inquire how progress made during the 'training' period compares with progress under conditions of 'practice'. In so doing, it should be remembered that the transfer question was the chief consideration when

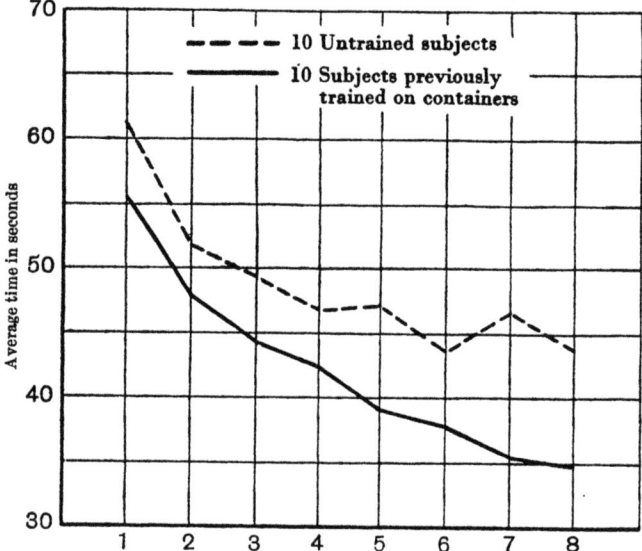

Fig. 46. Wedges operation. Practice graphs of trained and untrained groups of equal initial ability.

planning the training. Consequently, this was not arranged with a view to the development of maximum efficiency at the container operation *within the training period*. The scheme aimed at instruction and illustration rather than at speed. The operation as a whole was repeated only eighty-five times during the training period, as compared with the 440 times during practice. For these reasons, the training curve does not represent the efficiency that might have been attained, had the training aimed at the production of mere speed in the container operation itself by a judicious blending of 'practice' with instruction. At the same time, a comparison of the daily scores made by the trainees with those of the practisers is instructive, in showing the effect of substituting in large measure oral and visual instruction for mere repetition.

The relevant curves are given in fig. 47, where the deeper broken line indicates the daily scores of the 'practised' group and the other broken lines show those of various groups of 'trainees'. The latter are combined in the deeper continuous line which gives the average daily

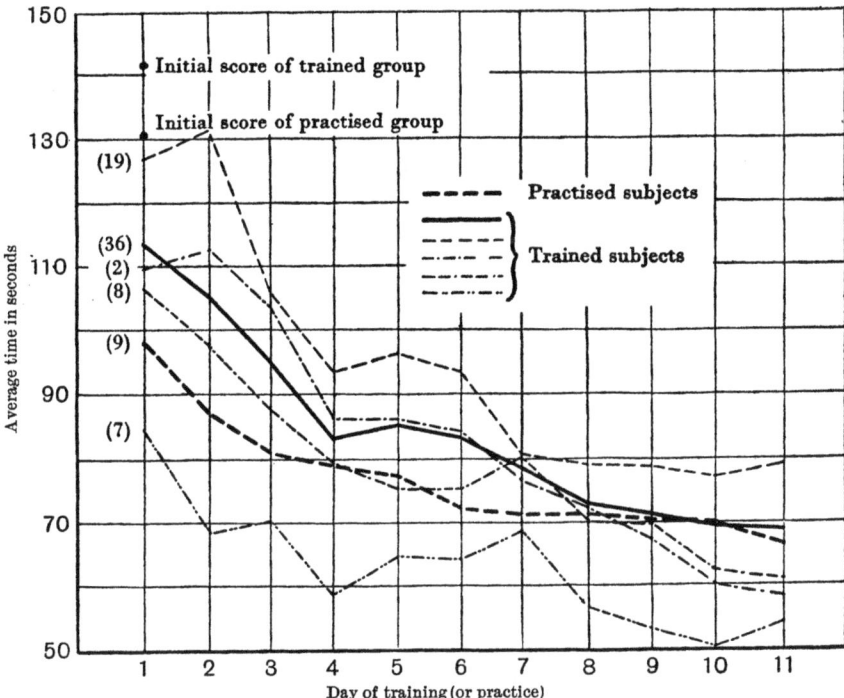

Fig. 47. Assembling containers. Comparison between practice and training curves. (Number of subjects in brackets.)

score for the whole thirty-six subjects. In every case the total progress of the trainees exceeds that of the practisers. A similar result is seen in the stripping curves, although in this simpler operation the difference between the two groups is less marked.

Fig. 48 shows similar data for groups starting initially equal, selected from the data of fig. 47, by pairing, as before, individuals initially equal. The additional practice gives the practised group the advantage at first; but by the eighth day the trainees have caught up to them. By this time, the practisers had repeated the operation 300 times, whereas the trainees had repeated it only forty times.

A similar result is seen in the curves for groups initially equal at stripping containers. In this simpler operation the rate of progress after the first day is much the same for both groups, but the trainees never quite recover from the advantage which the much larger number of repetitions gives to the practisers on the first day (forty repetitions as against one).

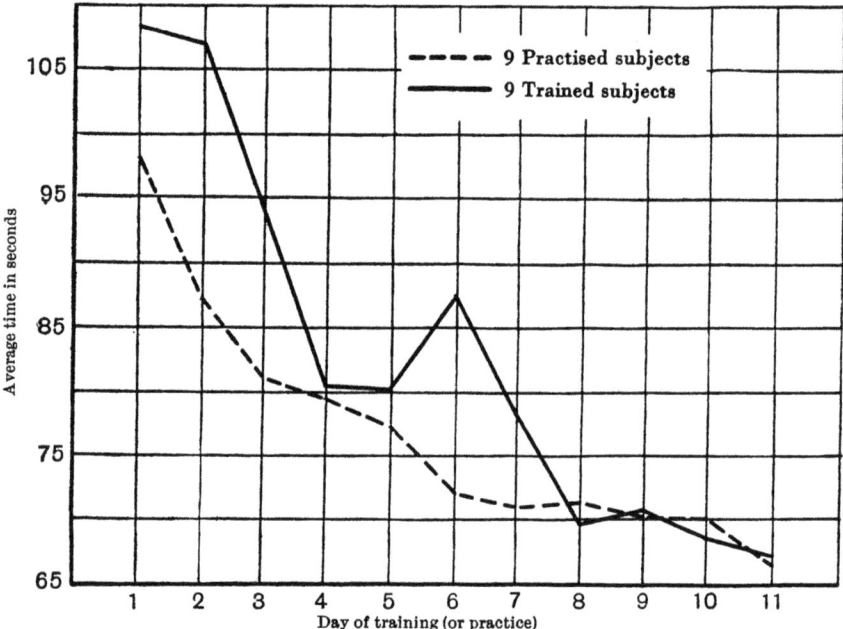

Fig. 48. Assembling containers. Comparison between practice and training groups.

(d) *The rôle of intelligence in 'training'.* It is an important practical consideration to ask how far the ability to profit by the training course may depend upon the trainee's general intelligence. This question has two aspects: (i) how far the ability to understand and apply the ideas during the training period was an expression of the subject's intelligence; and (ii) how far the ability to transfer and apply these ideas to the operation (wedges) which the trainees subsequently practised depended on their intelligence.

As regards the first question, all subjects took the test of the National Institute of Industrial Psychology for general intelligence

(Group Test 33). The correlations of this test with total progress made during the training period were as follows: with absolute improvement at assembling containers − 0·05, with absolute improvement at stripping containers − 0·41, with percentage improvement[1] at assembling containers 0·03, with percentage improvement at stripping containers − 0·38.

It is at once clear, from the absence of positive correlation, that general intelligence has played no large part in determining progress under training. It should be added that the negative coefficients must not be taken to imply that the possession of intelligence was a handicap to progress in the stripping operation. They are readily understood in the light of the relations which we have invariably found to hold in our numerous practised groups between these functions (intelligence and improvement) and *ability*. Whereas intelligence tends to a small positive correlation with the 'ability' which a subject initially displays at these operations, the ability itself tends to exhibit a marked negative correlation with the amount of improvement wrought by subsequent practice.[2] For this reason, we should expect intelligence likewise to exhibit a negative relationship with improvement.

To turn to the second question, the correlations of intelligence with the total progress made at the operations which the trained subjects subsequently practised were as follows: with absolute improvement at assembling wedges 0·15, with absolute improvement at stripping wedges − 0·16, with percentage improvement at assembling wedges 0·26, with percentage improvement at stripping wedges − 0·08.

Here, again, general intelligence can hardly be said to have been a serious determinant of progress, although it appears to have played a somewhat larger part than when directly applied to the training (in the container operation). Both here, and during the training period, the coefficients suggest the somewhat greater importance of intelligence in assembling than in stripping, and in 'training' than in 'practice'.[3] It was our aim to present the training ideas as simply and clearly as possible, and perhaps the most interesting indication given by these coefficients is the small part played by 'intelligence' in the assimilation and application of these ideas.

[1] I.e. the gain in time shown at the end of the training period over the initial score, expressed as a percentage of the initial score.
[2] Expressed differently, the higher one is on the scale of ability, the harder it becomes to make further progress.
[3] Having regard to the lower negative coefficients which were found for 'practice'.

D. CONCLUSIONS

Skill, developed by the mere repetition of one manual operation, confers little advantage in the performance of other operations that may be subsequently undertaken. Where, on the other hand, repetition is replaced by suitable instruction, the skill thus developed at no additional cost in time tends to transfer to other operations over a fairly wide range of manual activity. This transfer is manifested not only in superior ability, but also in a superior rate of progress. The advantage thus conferred by training was obtained, in the present experiments, without any loss of efficiency during the training period.

These results appear of great practical significance, wherever work requiring manual skill is involved, especially when it is remembered that the limits of proficiency to be attained by training may far exceed those attainable by uninstructed repetition. The results indicate the wastage that must be produced by the customary practice of allowing beginners in the assembly room to drop into the work as best they can. And they suggest that a very real advantage would follow from the replacement of this current crude procedure by a short course of systematic training in the general principles underlying manual control illustrated by specific examples from manual operations. A like procedure may be frequently adopted with advantage in other forms of manual activity, such as the work of our scholastic manual training centres, and 'coaching' for games, where often the so-called instruction offered resembles 'practice' rather than 'training'.

It is hardly necessary to add that, however important the effects of training may prove to be, they in no way negative the importance of inquiring into the effects of practice, for the two lines of inquiry, although similar, are not identical. What might have been transferred in 'practice' need not be the same as what actually was transferred in 'training'. A transference of practice effects would have suggested that the increased skill developed through practising one set of muscular co-ordinations had been transferred more or less directly to other series of co-ordinations in relative independence of the subjects' ideational activity. In other words, it would have suggested a transference on the neuro-muscular plane. The fact that no such transference was found, even in our more complex operations, suggests that the development of skill, when restricted to this neuro-muscular plane, is highly specific in its effects. On the other hand, consideration of the training scheme, and of the subjects' introspections, suggests that the transference in the 'training' experiments was effected at the ideational level, that there was no general change in the lower neuromuscular mechanisms but rather an increased facility in dealing mentally with situations that involve the use of the muscles concerned.

To discuss this question in relation to the general 'manual' factor which we found to run through these operations, and to 'general intelligence', would carry us beyond the scope of the present chapter. But, if we ask, in conclusion, how far this transference of ideas is one of innate general intelligence, and how far one of knowledge, wisdom or experience, the reply would seem to be the latter, since little correlation was found between general intelligence and the improvement, absolute or percentage, which the trainees subsequently made at the wedges operation. That this transference depends less on innate intelligence than on use of the knowledge acquired during training leads to the interesting corollary that training of this kind should be effective wherever there is present the modicum of intelligence needed to understand the simple ideas involved in the exercises.

PART IV

ANALYTICAL

CHAPTER XIV

SUBJECTIVE ANALYSIS OF 'MECHANICAL' ASSEMBLING

A. METHOD EMPLOYED

With a view to laying bare the mental processes involved in the 'mechanical' assembling tests (p. 31), detailed notes were made of the subject's behaviour while at work, and the subject's own introspective account of what had occurred mentally was taken down at the termination of each sitting. In making these observations our aim was to obtain, in as concise a form as possible, a complete record of the subject's actions during the test. Note was also taken of such indications of the subject's emotional and volitional reactions as might influence the result. To attain the necessary rapidity in writing, each of the parts to be assembled was referred to by letter.[1] Further abbreviation was rendered possible, after a while, by the fact that one became so familiar with certain constantly recurring features of the work that a single word, or a short phrase, was sufficient to record the whole situation. These notes were found useful not only in providing a permanent record for subsequent analysis, but in assisting the subject to recall certain points in his work upon which his introspection was sought and which would otherwise have been overlooked. This material, together with our own introspections, forms the basis of the subjective analysis which follows.

B. TWO SHARPLY DIFFERENTIATED ACTIVITIES

1. THE ACTIVITIES CONCERNED.

It will be remembered that in those which have been classified as 'mechanical' assembling tests, the subject was required both (i) to think

---

[1] The letters were those given in fig. 1 (p. 31).

out how the various parts should be fitted together to make the completed object, and (ii) to perform the actual task of fitting them together. It will be shown that the mental activity involved in (i) differs in many important respects from that in (ii). Consequently, it will make for clearness to consider, later on, each of these activities (hereafter called Activity I and Activity II) in turn. In doing so, however, we must avoid the impression that each necessarily runs its course in complete independence of the other. On the contrary, in the tests under consideration, the two kinds of activity are intimately related, both (*a*) temporally and (*b*) psychologically.

2. How related.

(*a*) *Temporally*. As regards the temporal relation of these two activities, a subject would seldom see how to assemble the whole object before he had assembled some of its parts. The usual course was to select certain parts which seemed to go together, fit these into the positions which they were thought to occupy, then make this the starting point for further work. If, as frequently happened, further progress in this direction was found impossible, the subject would turn to other parts. As a rule, it was only after trying several lines of attack, involving the active manipulation of the parts in a variety of ways, that the assembly was successfully completed. The two kinds of activity referred to thus proceeded in a series of closely interwoven steps. Some parts of the manipulative work would be sufficiently difficult to occupy the whole of the subject's attention.[1] Then of necessity it alternated with the task of discovering the positions of the parts in the completed object (Activity I). Other parts of this manipulative work were of a simple character, such as the picking up and turning over of a part, or the placing of one part beside, or inside, another. At these times the two kinds of activity appeared to proceed simultaneously, the manipulatory processes occupying the margin of consciousness, while those involved in thinking out the positions of the parts occupied its focus.

(*b*) *Psychologically*. The psychological relation between these two kinds of activity arises from the fact that the direction which one may take at any moment is apt to influence the direction taken by the other. For example, it frequently occurred that a subject would not realize

[1] For example, the screwing up of *E* (fig. 1) in the container test, that of *H* in the porcelain test, the threading of the wires through the holes in *M* and the subsequent screwing up of *K* in the wiring test.

the shape of the total solid made by parts B^1 when put together until, guided by the observed similarity in the shapes of their two flat surfaces, he had actually placed them with these surfaces coincident. The resulting shape was then observed and thus the way was opened to the next step, namely, the noting of the similarity between this shape and that of A. Many other instances could be given. In fact, it was the general rule to put together some of the parts first and then to modify subsequent work in the light of the observed result. The manipulation of the parts thus assisted the subject in much the same way as a figure helps one in geometry—by providing a means of apprehending and retaining relationships which, without these aids, the individual would find too complex to deal with.

Not always, however, did this handling of the material help forward the task. At times, it appeared to hinder progress.[2] This occurred in two circumstances. First, when certain of the parts were found to fit together in positions which they could not occupy in the finished object. For example, E could be (erroneously) screwed on to C by passing it over the top of C and screwing it downwards,[3] whereas the correct way was to pass it upwards over D and screw it upwards on C. When a false step of this kind had been made, the fact that the parts concerned did actually fit one another was apt to strengthen the subject's belief in the correctness of this step, and so lead to undue persistence in the wrong direction.

The second type of hindrance arose when certain of the parts had been correctly assembled, so far as their own relative positions were concerned, but with some of the 'intervening' steps omitted, so that it became necessary to undo these parts before the object could be completed. Typical examples were the screwing together of A and C with the wedges B left out (container test); the screwing of H into L before inserting the pin (I) and the spring (G) (porcelain test); attaching the wire to the porcelain (M) before slipping on C (wiring test). In cases of this kind, unlike those described in the previous paragraph, the hindrance arose not through persistence of effort in the wrong direction but through the loss of time consumed in unnecessary manipulation.

[1] The letters used throughout are given in fig. 1.

[2] 'Hinder', in the sense that time would have been saved if the steps here referred to had been avoided.

[3] The remainder of the assembly could not, of course, be completed with E in this position.

3. CONTINGENT NATURE OF THESE RELATIONS.

It should be noted that the above-described relations do not arise as a necessary consequence of the nature of the two activities concerned, but are contingent on the test and on the individual. Provided that the task is not beyond the power of the individual, there is nothing to prevent the whole of the 'thinking out' being done before handling a single part. Consequently, they throw little light on the psychological nature of the mental processes which constitute these activities, but are concerned with the courses which the two kinds of activity are observed to take. They have, however, an important bearing on the construction of this kind of test, as will be shown later.[1]

4. RELATIVE IMPORTANCE OF THE TWO ACTIVITIES.

Tests of 'mechanical' assembling are intended to measure, primarily, a person's ability to discover the positions occupied by the various parts in the completed object. Success or failure at the test should, therefore, turn upon this kind of activity rather than on the manipulative work that must of necessity be incurred in every assembling test. Especially is this so in view of the fact disclosed by our results, that each of these activities involves an independent factor[2] which cannot be measured in terms of the other. If the demand on manipulative skill is such as to influence seriously the subject's performance, the latter cannot be expected to afford a sound measure of the essential factor in 'mechanical' assembling.

We have seen that this factor is the same as that which enters as a special or 'group' factor in the mechanical aptitude tests.[3] Introspective observations indicate that the mental processes involved in the mechanical aptitude tests closely resemble those associated with Activity I in the mechanical assembling tests.[4] These facts, together with the additional circumstance that Activity II is entirely absent from the tests of mechanical aptitude, suggest that the specific correlation observed between these two groups of tests may be attributed to the common type, Activity I. Consequently, these specific correlations serve to indicate how far this kind of activity entered as a constituent in the mechanical assembling tests.

Similarly, some indication of the influence of Activity II is given by the specific correlations with the 'routine' assembling tests (p. 87),

[1] See p. 182.   [2] See p. 76.   [3] See p. 74.
[4] For the meaning of Activity I and Activity II see pp. 179, 182.

since in these the chief requirement was skill in manipulating the same material as was employed in the 'mechanical' assembling tests, Activity I being either entirely absent or reduced to a minimum. It must be remembered, however, that in this case the correlations illuminate only one aspect of the influence in question, namely, that associated with manipulative skill. Those other features of the manual work involved in 'mechanical' assembling to which we have referred above, were, of course, absent from the 'routine' tests.[1]

The necessary specific correlations were examined in Chapters VI and VII. They suggest that: (i) both the cognitive work involved in 'mechanical aptitude' (Activity I) and the manipulative skill involved in 'routine' assembling (Activity II) play a part in 'mechanical' assembling; (ii) with the exception of the 'tap' test (p. 38), the part played by the latter activity is small and decidedly less than that played by the former; (iii) the size of the specific correlation with mechanical aptitude varies directly as the complexity of the 'mechanical' assembling test, the order of complexity being 'porcelain', 'wiring', 'container', 'tap'. The last named, which was specially introduced on account of its simplicity, proves to be largely a test of manipulative skill. Its correlation with mechanical aptitude is negligible.

Hence follows the important suggestion that only the more complex objects are likely to provide useful material for tests of mechanical aptitude. Unless the task presented by the test is of sufficient difficulty, Activity I, which it is intended to measure, even when present, is apt to be masked by factors introduced by Activity II, the manipulative work, so that the score becomes a measure of the latter rather than of mechanical aptitude.

It is clear that of the two kinds of activity under discussion, that which is concerned with the solving of the problem, and which we have designated Activity I, is the one peculiar to 'mechanical' assembling as such, and that the activity involved in the *handling* of the material comes essentially to the 'front' in routine assembling. Consequently, we shall confine attention in the present section more especially to the mental processes in the former, and shall reserve our treatment of the latter for the section on routine assembling.

[1] At the same time, the specific correlation between the 'mechanical' and the 'routine' assembling tests must be partly explained by the mechanical factor (m), see p. 93.

C. GENERAL NATURE OF THE ACTIVITY PECULIAR TO 'MECHANICAL' ASSEMBLING

1. GENERAL OBSERVATION OF PARTS.

It will be remembered that the parts of the object to be assembled were spread on a sheet of paper in such a way that, when uncovered at the signal to begin, all were presented to view simultaneously. The subject's first step was to examine, more or less closely, the parts. This initial observation usually took the form of a general visual exploration of the whole before attempting to handle any, or to fit them together.

Its duration, as a distinct step, varied with the individual, and depended on: (i) the subject's previous knowledge, (ii) the nature of the knowledge acquired as the result of this general observation (to be considered hereafter), (iii) the speed of acquiring this knowledge, and (iv) certain temperamental qualities of mind which seemed to characterize the individual throughout the task. These appeared evident in this first step in the greater tendency of some persons to think ahead of their work and to see the consequence before putting any proposal into effect; whereas with others thought issued far more readily into action, so that the latter appeared to accompany and to illustrate the thinking rather than to follow from it. In no case, however, was this first step of long duration. It seldom, if ever, exceeded a minute, and usually occupied but a small fraction of this time; for as a rule a more or less cursory examination of the parts was sufficient to suggest how some of them might go, and the subject would then attempt to put into practice such ideas as occurred to him.

In spite of its brevity, this initial step was not without importance, for the mental work which was carried out during this short period, and which we have now to examine, sometimes greatly influenced the subsequent course of mental activity. Its importance is well illustrated in a short experiment which we performed with a few subjects, to see whether it was possible to employ this type of material in another fashion.[1] In this experiment the subject was asked to look carefully at the parts (without touching them) for one minute, and then, with the parts still before him, to answer questions as to where certain specified

[1] The method here suggested would have the advantage of presenting the problem in concrete form, without the complications arising from the practical manipulation of the material.

parts belonged in the completed object. One of these subjects re-marked that, in view of this experience, were he asked to do the assembling tests again, he would spend the first two or three minutes in carefully looking at the parts before attempting to assemble them.

2. First step: apprehension of simple attributes.

As the result of this initial exploration, the subject became aware of certain of the simpler attributes of the parts to be assembled; in particular, their shapes and sizes, and the sort of material of which they were made. With this knowledge came, (i) a recognition of the *general* purpose served by some of these parts, and (ii) a noticing of certain relations between these attributes. Of the parts whose *general functions* were thus immediately known, only three kinds entered into our tests, namely, the screw-threads on *K, H* and top of *C*, the threads on *A, F, E* and *L*, and the springs *G*. It remained, of course, a distinct problem at this stage to determine the special parts which these items played in the particular object to be assembled.

The relations observed at this stage were principally those of similarity, identity and difference. Thus, it was noticed at once that certain of the parts (those duplicated in the test material) were of the same shape, size and material (hence that there were 'two' of these): that these, again, differed in one or more of these respects from other parts; and that portions of the same 'part' were different in size or shape. Amid these differences there were observed, more or less immediately, certain points of resemblance—chiefly as regards 'shape' and 'number'. Thus such facts were noticed[1] as that the shape of the metal block *L* was similar to that formed by the curves of the **S**-shaped part of the porcelain piece *M*; that the 'number' of certain similar parts (such as *B, I, K, H, L* and *G*) was the same in each case ('two'), and similarly as regards the single pieces; that the holes in the porcelain (*M*) resembled the large screws (*H*) in number and size, and similarly as regards the small holes in *L* and the small screws (*K*). In like manner, the pieces *E* and *F*, although differing in one aspect of their shapes (their cross-sections) were similar as regards their both being 'rings', and of the same 'size'.

This initial step was referred to in the introspections of our subjects by such remarks as : "I was struck by the peculiar shape of the pieces

---

[1] With, at this stage, varying degrees of completeness and of clearness, to be remarked on presently.

of wood and wondered why they had this shape"; "I saw at once that there were a number of small pieces and a few larger pieces"; "I first looked carefully at the shapes of the pieces"; "I saw there were two of some pieces and only one of others"; "Seeing the spring, I concluded that it must fit into something in order to spring and be compressed". Further introspective reference to it will be found in our account of the second step. Its importance, however, was often overlooked in the introspections for the following reasons: (i) as a distinct step it was of short duration and still more so were the processes involved in it, being followed immediately by a much longer period of mental activity, it was apt to be forgotten by the time the test was finished; (ii) the subsequent mental work, dealing as it did with the real difficulties of the problem, was apt to obscure the importance of the initial observations, chief attention in the introspection being given to the subsequent activity; (iii) the concentrated effort involved in the latter was apt to inhibit memory of that which had immediately preceded it; (iv) some of the processes involved functioned in the margin of consciousness (or even subconsciously), and their consequent lack of clearness combined with their fleeting character to render them difficult of observation to any but trained introspectors; and (v) mental work of a similar, though usually more complex, character was continued in close association with the second step to which it immediately led, and from which, in consequence, it was not easily distinguished.[1]

3. SECOND STEP: ASSOCIATION OF PARTS 'MECHANICALLY'.

On the basis of such knowledge as we have described above, certain parts were associated together mentally as having some 'mechanical' connection with one another. The mental work involved here can best be described by an example. Let us suppose that the subject, as the result of the simple apprehension effected in the first step, has become aware (with varying degrees of clearness) of the sizes, shapes, colours, surface marks, and character of the material, of the parts (head and worm) of the screw H, and similarly as regards the metal block L, and of certain relations between these. The work of this present step consisted in associating together objectively certain of these parts (viz. the 'worm' and the 'hole') in the light of the observed relation ('simi-

---

[1] It is, of course, one thing to carry out a train of mental activity and quite another to observe what occurs mentally during the process—the mental processes in each case differ.

larity') between certain of their attributes ('size' and 'shape'). Thus, the observing of this similarity, conjoined with general knowledge as to how things behave, brought with it belief (with varying degrees of conviction) that (i) the screw would (or might) fit the hole, and (ii) that this might be its correct position in this particular object. As another example, we may consider the attempt made by many subjects to fit the springs (*G*) into the small holes of the block (*L*). Here the noting of the similarity between certain attributes of the spring (viz. 'size' and 'shape' of its cross-section[1]) and certain attributes of the small hole ('size' and 'shape' of its cross-section) led to the belief that the springs should be fitted into these holes—a belief which, in the light of subsequent activity yet to be described, proved erroneous. To take, finally, another case, the subject has recognized, by its shape and material, that *G* will behave as a spring and, likewise by its shape and material, that the hollow interior of *H* will act as a pocket; he now observes that this pocket will serve the purpose of holding one end of the spring steady while the other end 'springs'—in other words, in comparing the *behaviour* of the two pieces he is made aware of the *functional* relation one may bear to the other.

In general terms, then, the essential operation in this second step consists in observing that certain of the previously apprehended attributes are so related that the concrete parts which possess these attributes may stand in a 'mechanical' relationship towards one another. The attributes mainly concerned here were those of 'shape', 'size' and (to a less extent) 'number', together with those more complex attributes which are known by conjoining these presently apprehended attributes with past knowledge, and which we have called 'behaviour'[2] and 'function'—the latter being more complex than the former in that it involves, like the attribute 'behaviour', the reproduction of past knowledge—but this time as to how objects behave *towards one another*.

---

[1] Rarely of course, if ever, consciously expressed in these actual words in the subject's mind while carrying out the process itself.

[2] At this stage such knowledge of '*behaviour*' was of varying degrees of *generality*—from that of mere awareness of the general physical properties of the part, to a more particularized knowledge of the general purpose served by it—its 'mechanical' behaviour. Only one other form of particularized knowledge was observed, viz. 'aesthetic' behaviour, and that on only one occasion, when a subject observed that he was partly guided in putting the ring *F* on *D* by the thought that it gave a "finished appearance" to the object. It is noteworthy that this was the only piece in our tests which possessed no 'mechanical' function, and it was on this account omitted from our subsequent work with the elementary school groups.

It remains to explain how, from the observance of the relations between certain of the apprehended attributes, the thinking of the parts as being *'mechanically'* connected comes about. Why, for example, does the subject connect[1] the spring *G* with the pin *I*, or with the screw *H*, or (erroneously *in the present test*) with the small hole in *L*, rather than with the small screw *K* which it also resembles in some respects, but with which it was never connected? Here, again, the basis of such thinking lies partly in the subject's past experience, by which it is known that one connection is more probable than another, and partly in the closeness and number of the relations observed between the parts concerned. Thus *G* is related to *I* both in size, shape and function, whereas to *K*, merely in certain very limited aspects of its size and shape—*K* when screwed into *G* fulfilled no conceivable purpose.[2]

Finally, we come to the 'mechanical' relatedness to which we have referred, and which becomes known as the result of this kind of thinking. By this we mean the particular relation in which each part must be placed with regard to the others in order that it may fulfil the purpose required of it in the completed mechanism. To attain to this knowledge with respect to all the parts was the essential problem of the test. Such complete knowledge was not, of course, obtained in this second step.[3] On the contrary, much more mental work was needed to bring to full awareness all the connections necessary to the complete solution of the test. Such connections as were observed were usually thought of as being merely 'probable' or 'possible'. These, however, provided the starting point for the subsequent work. The following introspective observations refer to the work of this step: "I decided from their shapes (apprehended in first step) that the larger pieces must form the outer portion of the lampholder while the smaller piece must somehow be attached to the porcelain"; "I noticed there were screws (appre-

---

[1] In the sense of being functionally associated in the object to be assembled.

[2] For this reason it is probable that the weak relation between *G* and *K* was not even noticed by the testee, for, as we shall see later (p. 209), the mental activity is guided throughout by *purpose* and is, on this account, *selective*.

[3] Except in a few instances with the 'wiring' test. This differed from the 'porcelain' and 'container' tests in that, strictly speaking, it required the working out of only one (complex) mechanical relationship, viz. that between the wire and the lampholder, the mode of assembling the latter being already known. It also differed in that it was necessary to think out the complete manner of attaching the wire before its attachment could be *correctly* begun, whereas certain parts of the other tests could be correctly assembled without reference to the remaining parts.

hended in first step), so I looked for holes into which these would fit"; "I connected the two pins (apprehended in first step) with the two holes (apprehended in first step) in the blocks".

4. THIRD STEP: FURTHER CONFIRMATION, CLARIFICATION, AND DEVELOPMENT OF THOUGHT.

As we have already hinted, the knowledge acquired so far was usually lacking in completeness and certainty.[1] Nevertheless, it was sufficient to provide the starting point for a more or less systematic attempt[2] to fit the parts together. Having decided how certain parts might fit together, the subject now picks up these parts and attempts to assemble them in the way in which the mental work already described has led him to think they go. This constitutes the beginning of the third step.

Success in these attempts tended to confirm belief in the correctness of his method, whereas failure usually led to the conviction that the parts in question could not, after all, be connected in the way they were thought to be. Such confirmation or denial was not always justified; as, for example, where subjects screwed, quite successfully but erroneously, the ring E over the part C, or when, having passed screw H through the hole in the porcelain, they failed through lack of dexterity to get it to 'bite' on to the hole in the block L. Here we have interesting examples of the instrusive influence of Activity II on the course of the processes involved in Activity I. Incidentally, they illuminate the problem of test construction—a matter to which we shall return later.

As the manipulation of the various parts continued, it was accompanied by a closer examination of the parts themselves. Those which had not been 'mechanically' connected hitherto now received special consideration. They were twisted and turned in various directions, and placed in close juxtaposition to one another and to such parts as had been already put together, with a view to discovering how all might be incorporated into a single object. This more careful looking at the parts from all aspects brought to clearer apprehension many attributes which had been overlooked hitherto.[3] Among such may be

---

[1] As denoted by such introspection as: "I wondered whether the pieces of wood would fit on top of the cap, and whether the grooves in them fitted into the projections".

[2] In contrast to mere 'trial and error'.

[3] As expressed by one subject: "I suddenly saw that the shape of the block fitted into that of the porcelain. I did not notice this for a long time".

cited, as chief examples, the small metal projections at the top of C, the kinks in the base of C and in D, the flanges at the ends of the pins I, the grooves in the wooden wedges B, and more precise knowledge of the sizes and shapes of the holes in the porcelain M and in the blocks L. Thereupon, followed a further awareness of relations. This came about in two ways, namely (i) by comparing certain of these newly apprehended attributes with one another, or with those which had been already observed, and (ii) by observing the results of the attempts to fit certain parts together, which were made in consequence of these observations, in the way that we have already described.

Examples of (i) were the space relation ('opposite') between the two kinks on the base of C; that between the kinks on D; the 'identity' of these two relations[1] (leading to the placing of the two parts so that the kinks on one corresponded with those on the other); the functional relation between the grooves on the wedges and the projections on C; and more detailed knowledge of the space relations between the holes in M, and between those in L. Examples of (ii) were the clearer knowledge of the space relations which H would bear to L when assembled, which came through actually screwing H into L, and which, in turn, afforded some indication of the function of H; the quantitive relation between the length of wire left protruding through the top of the lampholder (C) and the distance through which it had to pass in order to reach to L, and which often led to better judgment, in subsequent wiring tests, as to the amount which should be left protruding; and the space relations between the holes in L and those in M, which obtained when L was actually placed in M, and which led to knowledge as to which side uppermost L should be placed.

It is clear that the mental processes here are similar to those of the preceding steps, but are now carried out on the basis of the wider experience which comes from the practical manipulation of the parts. In consequence, knowledge (of certain attributes[2]) which had been previously lacking, or had been obscure and incomplete, now attains to greater clearness and completion. Thought thus underwent a process of *clarification*.

In another way, too, the attributes differed from those dealt with in

---

[1] Expressed in the introspections as noticing that the positions of the kinks on C corresponded (or were similar) to those of the kinks on D.

[2] Such attributes include, technically, both characters, such as 'shape' and 'size', and the relations between these.

the former steps, namely, in their greater *complexity*. Thus the subject would usually observe, without much difficulty, that the screw H screwed into the block L and that the spring G fitted into the pin I. It required more thinking to discover that the pin, together with its accompanying spring, must be placed through the large hole of L before screwing on H—and yet more to discover that, in order to attach these to the porcelain, the screw should be put through the large hole in the latter before being screwed on to L. To pass over these customary stages in the solution of this test the mind was called upon to deal with relations of continually increasing complexity. Thus, in the last and critical stage the subject had to keep in mind not only the interrelation of G, I and L, but also the relations between these and the screw H and the porcelain M.

A further characteristic feature of this step was the increasing directional influence which knowledge already acquired (during the course of assembling) exerted on the work yet to be carried out. For example, the subject would first discover that G would go inside I and that I would fit into L; H would then be screwed on to L not merely on account of its observed relation to this piece, but also because it would hold I and G suitably in place. Similarly, the wedge B would at times be assigned to its right place, not primarily because of its observed relation to A, but because this seemed the only suitable place in the light of the knowledge gained in assembling all the other parts. In these cases, the previously cognized items seem to fuse together and to function as a whole. It is clear that such fusion is correlative to their above-described complexity, so that both may be regarded as complementary phases in a single developmental process. In this way, thought is seen to undergo much further *development* during the course of this third step.

5. Fourth step:

(*a*) *Active search.* Knowledge of all the 'mechanical' relationships which enter into the problem may become clear by the processes already described, in which case the test terminates with the third step. More frequently, however, after the subject had 'mechanically' connected as many parts as he could in this way, there still remained certain more difficult connections to be discovered, which constituted the crucial problem, or *pons asinorum*, of the test. In the porcelain test, for example, the parts G, I, L and H were usually assembled together in the manner we have been considering. It remained then a distinct problem to determine how this portion could be attached to the porcelain part, and one which often provided great difficulty. In the container test a crucial problem was the way of fixing together C and D; and, to a less extent, the method of assembling the wedges B. In the wiring test it proved sometimes to be the mode of attaching the wire to the block L.

The mental work involved here differed from that which characterized the foregoing steps, in that it now consisted of an *active search* for a solution to a clearly defined problem, during which mental processes essentially different from those so far described might be employed. This, together with the more intense feelings of perplexity with which it was usually associated, suggest its separate consideration as a fourth step. At the same time, it should be observed that it was not impossible to effect this work by means of the processes already described; nor were the processes we are about to consider always absent from the third step. In general, however, the earlier and easier connections were discovered by the processes constituting the third step, while the working out of the solution to the more difficult problem which then usually remained over lent itself more especially to the kind of process now to be described.

This may best be made clear by an account of what frequently happened with the container test. In the light of observed relationships between their shapes, the subject has fitted B into A, and A on to C, and has discovered the correct position of C with respect to D—all of which constitute the third step. The problem which remains for solution, and which is now clearly framed in his mind, is how to join C to D—a problem which, in spite of its apparent simplicity, often gave considerable trouble. He *may* solve it in the following manner. Holding the larger rim of C against that of D, he notices that the latter curves outwards to meet the edge of C. He is also aware of the screw-thread on the rim of C and of the space relations between the two rims. From these observations he concludes that the thing required is a ring which will overlap both rims, screw on to C and curve inwards over D. Consequently, he looks for a ring with a curved edge, chooses E (rather than F), and correctly assembles it (i.e. over D rather than over C).

This process differs fundamentally from those previously considered; for, whereas in the previous steps the part is first presented to the mind and is then assembled in the light of its subsequently cognized attributes, in the present step there is first awareness of the required attributes (arising from knowledge as to where the part must go, or what it must do, as formulated in the problem) from which follows the selecting of the part possessing these attributes. Knowledge as to which part did in fact possess the required attributes may be already known from previous observations. This was usually so in the above-cited example. On the other hand, the required part was at times only found after much further search. In this, however, the mental work was essentially of the same character as that of the earlier steps, but also included simple recognition of the attributes, when found, as being those sought for in the part. Such further search was frequently observed in the porcelain test. Here the problem was rendered more difficult because: (i) the problem was itself less clearly defined, for the subject was not always sure that the parts concerned had to be attached to the porcelain; (ii) the attributes sought in the required part were less restricted in character, for there was some scope for variation in the manner of attaching the parts; and (iii) they were of greater complexity, for they included as their primary constituents the somewhat intricate space and functional relations which the screw H was required to bear to the porcelain and to the other parts.

(*b*) *Alternative procedures.* We have already remarked on the conditions under which this fourth step did not appear as a distinguishable phase. This occurred when the work of the third step left nothing further to be done. It remains to be added that when this was not the case the ensuing work was not invariably carried out in the above-described way. This happened when (i) the subject was unable to formulate with sufficient clearness and precision the problem which remained for solution, or (ii) when he found it impossible to cognize the attributes involved in the solution of this problem. In neither case was there sufficient knowledge of what to look for to render a search possible.

Two alternative procedures were then possible. One of these consisted essentially in a continuance of the same sort of mental work as that of the third step. The parts remaining to be assembled were compared with each other, and with the work already done, in various positions, and such 'mechanical' connections as suggested themselves in the light of these comparisons were tried out until all the remaining parts had been assigned to their correct positions. For reasons given in our last paragraph it was the method which weaker subjects were more likely to adopt. Its shortcomings were clearly seen in the container test where, owing to their close resemblance in shape, the ring *E* was frequently placed over *C*—an error which sometimes led to much loss of time.

The other alternative more nearly approached that of pure 'trial and error'.[1] Here the attempts to complete the assembling were guided not so much by any observed attributes as by the hope that one of the various positions in which the parts were tried would prove to be correct. The knowledge by which its correctness was recognized came *after* the trial rather than before it.

There were observed three varieties of this method which, we suggest, may be distinguished by the adjectives 'systematic', 'random', and 'unconscious', respectively.

In the systematic type, the part (or parts) is thought to occupy one of certain positions which are tried *in turn*. An example was furnished by the connecting together of *C* and *D*. Here the problem was to know which of two rings to use, and which of two ways to put it on. Each of these four possibilities was tried in turn without reference to the peculiarities on the shapes of the rings or to the functions which the peculiarities serve, such as is required in the method of 'search'.

The 'random' variety of 'trial and error' may be illustrated by the same piece of work. In this, knowledge did not proceed so far as to systematize the possibilities, but only so far as to recognize the probability that the two pieces were connected by a ring, whereupon the ring and the position in which it is tried were selected at random.

The 'unconscious' kind occurs when the 'trial' itself is performed unconsciously while the mind is engaged on something else. This happened with some frequency in assembling the wedges *B*. These would be placed in *A*, and the latter would then be screwed on to the top of *C*. During the course of the screwing the grooves in the outer sides of the wedges would sometimes fall into place on the projections in the top of *C* without the subject realizing that these existed. Similarly, the existence and function of the kinks on *D* and *C* were at times only

---

[1] 'Pure' because the 'trial' is in no wise guided by insight into the conditions which govern its success (in the present case, the 'mechanical' characters and relations) and to distinguish it from much so-called 'trial and error' in which such insight is not entirely lacking, but is merely obscure and incomplete.

observed after the groove on the porcelain *M* had accidentally fallen into its correct position during the screwing up of *E*.

Although these 'trial and error' methods did not play a large part in the present tests, they illuminate the problem of test construction, for clearly any test which aims at measuring the processes peculiar to assembling should not be capable of solution too readily by methods of 'trial and error'.

D. THE COGNITIVE PROCESSES IN 'MECHANICAL' ASSEMBLING

1. MEANING OF TERMS.

Having reviewed the principal operations involved in 'Intelligent' assembling, we are now in a position to enumerate, by way of summary, the cognitive processes upon which success at this kind of work essentially depends. For this purpose, it will be necessary to employ certain technical terms[1] which, for the convenience of those who may be unfamiliar with them, we will first explain, using for this purpose examples from our tests.

(*a*) *Apprehension of experience.* As example, let us suppose the various parts to be assembled are placed before the subject for the first time. As soon as he brings his mind into relation with any of them (in the present test by looking at them) he tends to know *immediately*, i.e. without the intervention of any other mental process, *something* of the resulting experience. The mental process by which this immediate knowing comes about is called 'apprehension'. It should be noted that it is a knowing of something given in the experience itself, such as the shape of the head of screw *H*, which results from looking at it, and is not to be confused with knowledge which may be inferred from this by conscious association with knowledge already in the mind and now recalled; as, for example, the shape of the rest of the screw which may now be inferred from the present apprehension of its head, i.e. without the rest actually being looked at, provided the subject is already possessed of sufficient knowledge about such screws.

(*b*) *Characters.* The *something* about the experience which is known by apprehension and which is referred to above in italics, is known as a *character*. Thus the above-mentioned shape of the head of *H* is

---

[1] For a full account of these see C. Spearman, *The Nature of 'Intelligence' and the Principles of Cognition* (London: Macmillan, 1923).

termed a character of that head. Other characters are its size and its solidity.

Characters may be apprehended with varying degrees of *clearness*. Thus the *shape* of the above screw was clearly known, while its *weight* was but obscurely apprehended, if at all, for it played no part in the problem.

(*c*) *Eduction of relations*. Having apprehended two (or more) characters, such as the *shape* of screw *H* and *shape* of the hole in block *L*, a further mental process is now possible, namely, an immediate awareness of the *relation* ('similarity') between them. This process is known as 'eduction'. As in the case of 'apprehension', the knowledge of relations which comes by eduction is generated immediately from the presented 'characters'. It must be distinguished from similar knowledge which may be arrived at indirectly. Thus, the above-mentioned 'similarity' may be known by inference from knowledge that the screw must fit the hole, or by recall, or simply from report, in which cases the related characters (shapes) need not be presented mentally, or even known.

(*d*) *Fundaments*. The items between which a relation is reached or 'educed' are termed its 'fundaments'. Thus, the above-mentioned shapes of *H* and the hole respectively are the fundaments of the relation 'similarity'. Not only characters but also relations may serve as fundaments, as when our subjects saw that the space relation which one screw *H* bore to one block *L* was *similar* to that borne by the other screw *H* to the other block *L*. Here the fundaments are the two space relations, and the educed relation is that of similarity. From such simplicity they may attain to great complexity. A more complex instance occurs when it is seen that the relation which the small screws *K* bear to the blocks *L* is different from that which the large screws *H* bear to the same blocks. Here the fundaments from which is educed the relation of *difference* are themselves complex relations.

It is important from the point of view of test construction and analysis to notice that a character or relation need not, from the mere fact of its being presented mentally, become a fundament generating further knowledge. This will only occur when the above-described process of 'eduction' takes place. Thus, in our previously quoted example, it is conceivable that the *weight* of the screw *H* might be noticed by an individual who, expecting to pick up a solid screw, found it lighter than he anticipated. This item would thus become an apprehended character of the screw.[1] As it was immaterial to the solving of the test, this would hardly be related to any other character, and so would not be likely to function as a fundament. Quite different would have been the case if the test had been so arranged that the weight of the assembled object mattered, and the subject had to choose between a variety of screws of different weight. Although this may appear very obvious, it illustrates a point often overlooked in introspective work, namely, that it is not enough to know merely what passes before the mind, but rather how these mental occurrences function, and how relevant to the success of the work such functioning is.

(e) *Eduction of correlates.* Let us suppose that there is presented mentally any character such as the *length* of a given screw, together with a relation such as *twice.* Then it is possible to know directly from these two given items a second character which bears that relation to the given length. This newly generated character is known as a 'correlate'. Again the process is one of eduction, since this knowledge of the correlative character is derived immediately from the initially known character and relation. As before, the given character and the educed correlate are termed fundaments, and not only characters but also relations may function as either fundament. An illustration of the latter occurred in the porcelain test, where, after having discovered how to assemble one-half of the object, the subject could straightway assemble the other. Here the given (complex) fundament is supplied by the *space relations* between the various parts of the first half; the given relation which these space relations are known to bear to those between the parts of the second half is that of *identity*, whence the immediately known space relations between the parts of the second half constitute the educed correlate. The whole process is represented in fig. 49; the spatial characters ('shape' and 'size') of the parts by squares, the relations (space) between them by circles, the given fundament and relation which function in the process, described above, by thick unbroken lines, the educed correlate by thick dotted lines. The same figure indicates the complexity of the fundaments in this instance; involving not less than fifteen relations. It also serves to illustrate what is meant by their functional character, for while all these relations are *known*, in the sense of being intended and meant

[1] Apprehended, of course, with varying degrees of *clearness* according to the person's ability to estimate weight, and according to its position with respect to the focus of consciousness.

when the eductive process takes place, they are not necessarily all in consciousness, much less in the focus of consciousness, at the moment when the eductive process occurs.

(*f*) *Attributes*. To avoid more technical language we have already used the term 'attribute'. This may be defined as anything that is known of anything else. Its denotation includes, and is covered by, the above-mentioned characters and relations.

(*g*) *Reproduction*. This term will be employed in its usual meaning to denote the process whereby any known attribute may be recalled to

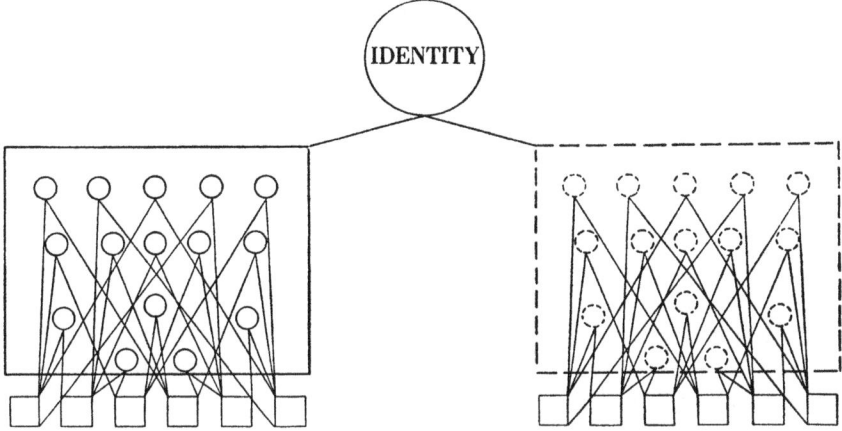

Fig. 49. Diagrammatic representation of mental processes involved in cognizing the second half of the porcelain mechanical assembling operation.

mind. Introspection indicates that the recalled items—known as 're-products'—may vary in clarity and complexity in the same way as do educed items ('educts').

2. THE ESSENTIAL PROCESSES.

(*a*) *Apprehension*. (i) *The characters apprehended*. Reverting to the work of 'mechanical' assembling, it is clear that the initial processes were those defined above as apprehensive, and the characters to be apprehended were chiefly those of 'shape' and 'size'. In the material of the present tests, these characters were sufficiently simple to suggest that their clear apprehension under appropriate psychological conditions was well within the capacity of all our subjects. Hence, while being an essential preliminary to the work which was to follow, this initial apprehensive work was not, generally speaking, the chief determinant of success or failure at the test as a whole.

(ii) *Psychological conditions for their apprehension.* The more obvious of these characters came readily to view in what we have referred to as the first step of the work. Usually, however, as we have already seen, the apprehension of less obvious characters continued, more or less, throughout, and some of these were, at times, entirely overlooked by weaker subjects. Since knowledge of these had an important bearing on the method of assembly, the psychological conditions under which they came to clear apprehension is not without interest. In view of their relative simplicity, the determining factor, in the present instances, appears to be the *direction* taken by attention. This itself seems to depend on two further factors: (i) the indication given by the items already cognized, and (ii) the natural tendency for the mind to notice more readily that with which it is already familiar. A person, for example, familiar with the use of 'kinks' and 'flanges' and specially shaped screwheads, would be more apt to notice these in consequence. This latter factor raises the question, important for test construction and interpretation, as to the sort of characters which, when introduced into a test, may favour those who have had special training.

(iii) *Apprehension of complex shapes.* Regarding the former factor—the direction of attention by previously cognized items—this would seem to be more closely associated with innate ability. As such, it seemed worth while attempting to inquire more closely into the psychological processes underlying the cognizing of shape. From observations on our subjects it seemed clear that fuller knowledge of the shape of any given part might arise in two conversely related ways. It might come by the subsequent conjoining of two or more separately apprehended characters into a single shape. For example, it would sometimes happen that first the 'roundness' of ring E would be apprehended, and then the 'curvature' of the edge. Conversely, it seemed sometimes that the shape as a whole was first apprehended—as, for example, that of pin I—whence certain details, such as that of the flange on the pin, subsequently emerged. Both cases are readily explained by the facts that (i) the shape of the whole part is itself a complex character made up of simpler characters (such as the above-mentioned 'roundness' and 'curvature'); and (ii) the method by which the whole shape comes to be clearly apprehended depends on the way attention is directed to these more elementary constituents. What the shape gains in extensity when apprehended as a whole it evidently loses in clearness.

Closely associated with this question is the observation, made by some subjects, that they had great difficulty in cognizing the shape that would be formed by putting together mentally the two wedges *B* as they go when assembled. For this reason they failed to associate the wedges with the piece *A* into which they fit. In these cases what seemed to be known clearly were (i) the shape of each separate wedge, and (ii) their spatial relation when put together. The difficulty experienced by these subjects may be more clearly understood if we realize that it was evidently not one of *knowing all about* the resulting shape, since (i) and (ii) alone provide all the knowledge needed to locate every point in space either within or on the surface of the resulting solid, and all the space relations between these points. It is evident that all this may be known without knowing the shape itself. It may be compared with the kind of knowledge of the spatial character of a country that is got by walking over it without ever seeing a map of it. Clearly, what these subjects failed to do was to apprehend as a *single whole* the shape of the solid which would be made by placing the separate pieces into the given space relation.

Further light on the nature of this process was shed by observations on children. In these, owing to its less developed state, the process could be better examined in relation to simpler shapes, and without the complications introduced by three dimensions. A number of simple geometrical designs composed of straight lines and simple curves, such as could be immediately apprehended by most adults, were presented in turn to each of the two lowest classes of a girls' elementary school[1] (children aged 7–8 years). The children were asked to look carefully at the design and draw exactly what they saw—the copy remaining before them. When their efforts were examined, it was seen that, while all the lines were invariably put in, the space relations between them which determined the shape of the design were frequently overlooked. One of the most interesting cases observed was the copy of a mechanical diagram made by a girl of 6 years 7 months[2] at her own request. It is shown in fig. 50. The noteworthy feature is the position given to the spokes in wheel *B*. Thinking that such a result might be due to carelessness, the writer asked the child to look at her drawing of the wheel and say whether she thought it was right. At first she replied "Yes"; then, on being further questioned whether there was anything wrong with the spokes, she said with a crestfallen air, "Yes, I couldn't get eight spokes in—there are eight in your drawing". Now it is not suggested that this child could not see that the spokes met at the centre

---

[1] The same that had provided our older girl subjects.

[2] Not a member of the above class, but my own daughter, Karin.

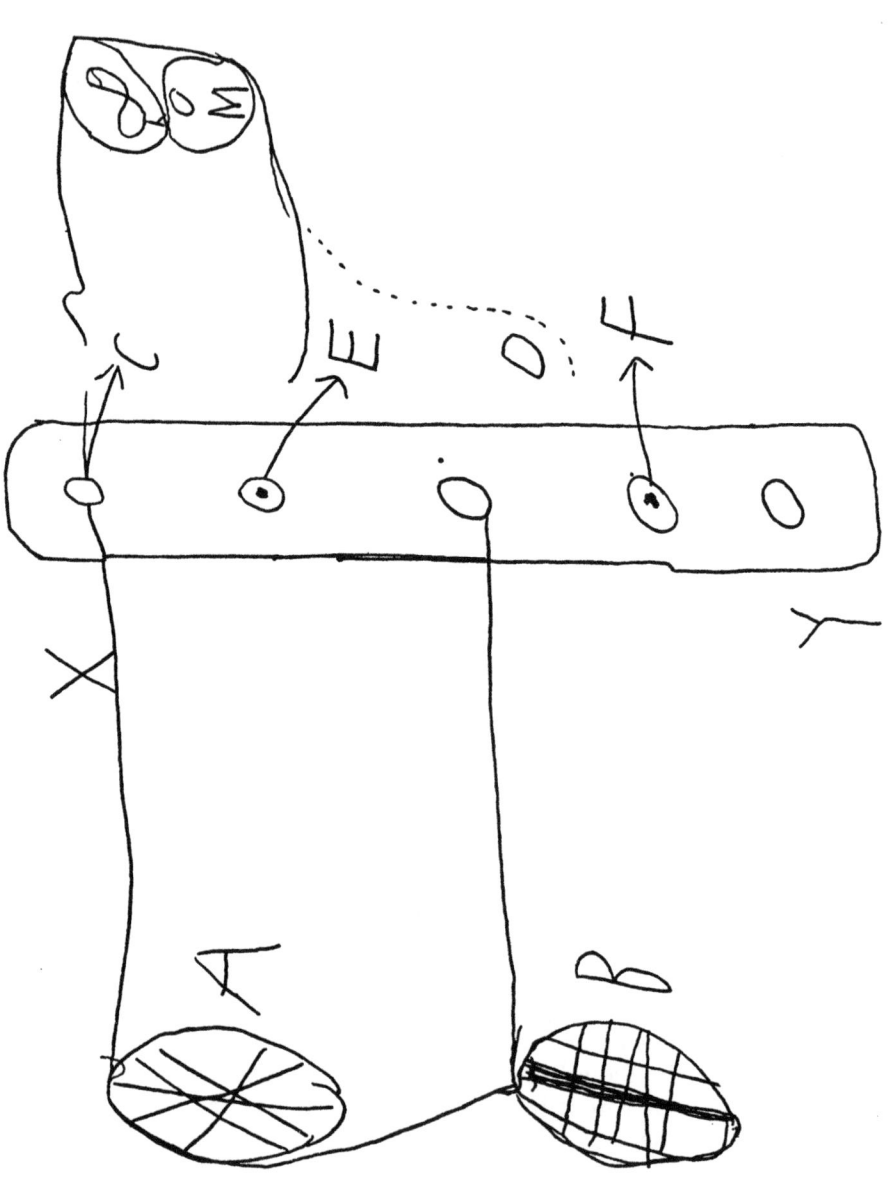

Fig. 50. Copy of a mechanical diagram made by a girl aged six years and seven months. (*Reduced.*)

of the wheel, or that such knowledge was necessarily entirely lacking. What does seem evident is that the space relations between the spokes and rim were far less clearly cognized than were the shapes of the spokes and rims themselves, so that in the child's efforts to get their number right she failed to observe their space relations, or to remember them while drawing.[1] A further indication of this appeared in the fact that, both here and in the above-mentioned designs, the number of such symmetrically repeated items was got not by drawing them first in their correct relationships, as would almost certainly be done by an adult subject, but by counting them. The average adult would usually draw the spokes correctly without realizing their number. All this goes to show that the child mind does not apprehend these more complex shapes as single immediately known *wholes*, as the adult tends to do, and that such failure is due to difficulty in cognizing the space relations between the parts.

An interesting example from everyday life has been furnished the writer by Dr C. S. Myers, who recounted to him that native adults, on observing a picture that was being painted in Cairo by a friend of his, were heard to exclaim: "Look, there's a window—there's a door—there's a chimney—why, it's a house". Fig. 51 shows an attempt to copy a flower, made by the child aged 6 years and 7 months, to whom we have already referred, and fig. 52 shows her four successive attempts to draw a cup standing on a saucer. In both, the inability to grasp the space relations between the elementary shapes which constitute the whole is clearly evidenced.

(b) *The fundamental questions.* We have seen that the real difficulty in the tests was to discover the relative positions which the various pieces occupy in the completed object. Here the task differs from that of apprehending shapes, in that in the latter the relations between the more elementary characters constituting the whole complex shape are given in the shape itself, whereas now they have to be invented. To bring out the difference in another way, we may compare the apprehension of the shape to the cognizing of a given design, whereas the task we have now to examine is akin to that of constructing the design itself. Unlike our former lines and circles, the parts constituting this 'design' are three-dimensional, somewhat irregular, shapes, and the conditions which the design must fulfil are mechanical rather than geometrical.

[1] She drew with the copy before her.

Here, as in all other designing, various possible relationships into which the elements (the pieces to be assembled) may be placed must first be considered; and from these must be chosen those relationships which fulfil the purposes of the design. In the present instance, the 'design' was known as a lampholder; but it was often less determinately known as merely 'a definite object in which all the given parts fit together'. It is clear that without this limitation of purpose quite other relationships could be selected to make, with the same

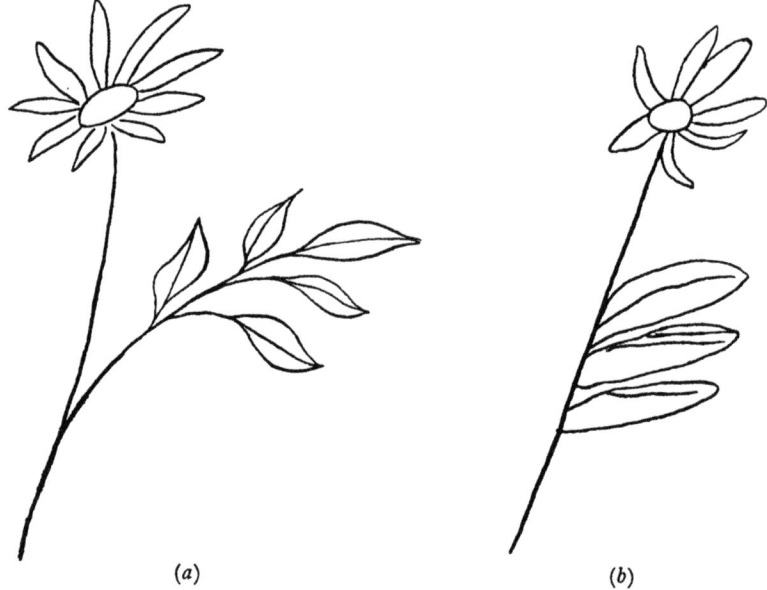

(a)   (b)

Fig. 51. The copy (b) made of the flower (a) by a girl aged six years and seven months.
(*Reduced.*)

parts, other 'designs'; as, for example, 'the most artistic arrangement of the parts on the paper'. The extent to which other possibilities are likely to be considered will not, of course, always be the same in respect of any two parts. It will depend on (i) whether the correct relationship between them is already known, either before the test begins or from knowledge which has been acquired about other parts while the test is in progress, and (ii) the indications afforded by the character of the parts themselves. Thus, when once the similarity between the two halves of the porcelain and the position of one H screw is known, the position of the second H screw is known; and the

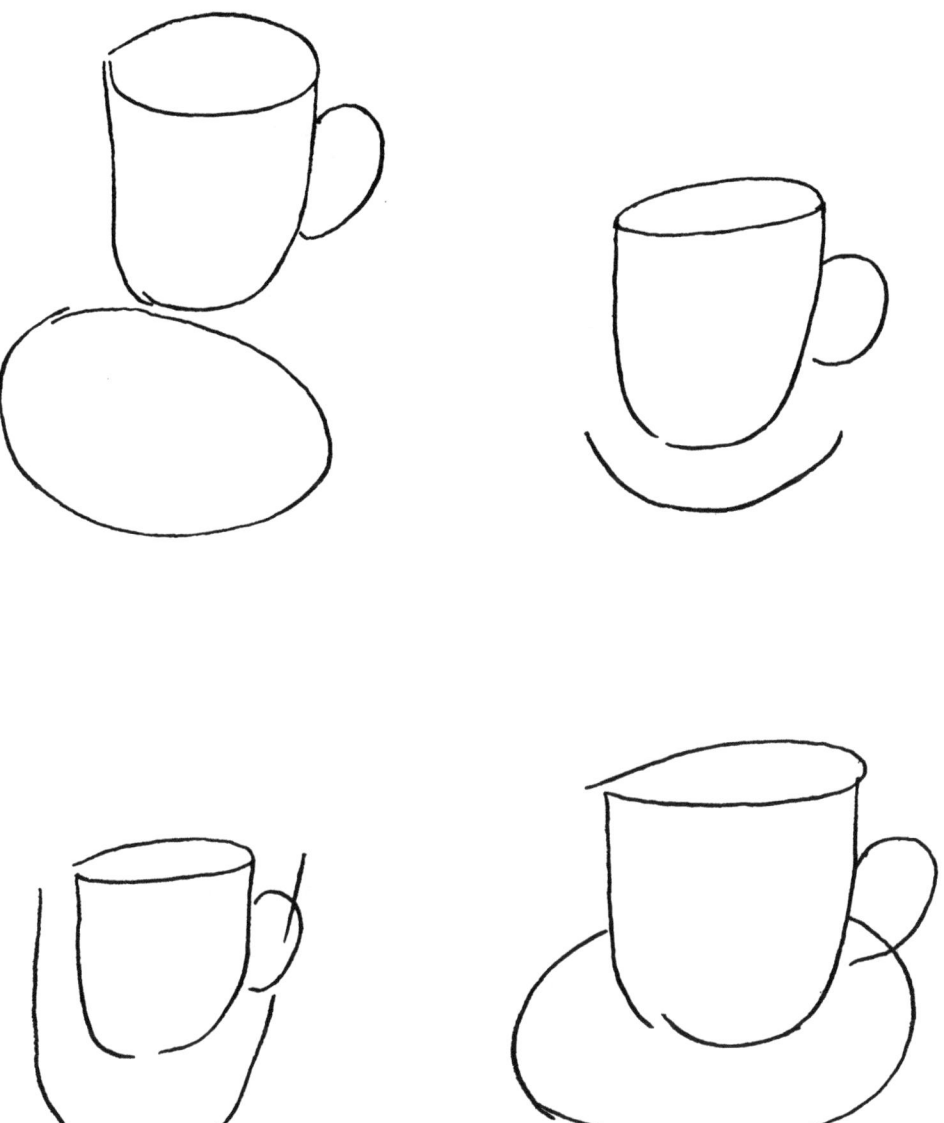

Fig. 52. Four successive attempts to draw a cup and saucer by a girl aged six years and seven months. (*Reduced.*)

characters of ring E (shape, size and thread) indicate, within very narrow limits, its relation to the other parts.

The two fundamental psychological questions, then, are firstly how do these *possible* relations become known, and secondly, how from these are the *right* ones discovered. The first seems concerned more closely with what is commonly called 'fertility of ideas', the second with 'critical power'.

(c) *Eduction of relations between characters.* Regarding the first of these questions, in so far as the relations are not indicated by work already done on the test, or recalled from previous experience, the process by which they become known is that of 'eduction'. In this the apprehended characters of all parts function as fundaments between which *may* be educed an infinite variety of relations. The number and kind that *are* actually educed are, of course, limited by the general nature of the problem as cognized by the subject before he begins his task.

(i) *The characters.* In the present tests, the characters functioning as fundaments were principally those of 'shape', less focally 'size' and, to a more limited extent, 'number' and 'function'. Concerning 'shape', it was seldom the whole shape, but usually one or more of its elementary characters, which functioned as the fundaments. Thus, in noting the resemblance between the shape of block L and part of porcelain M, the fundaments were not the whole shapes of these parts but of certain of their elementary constituents, namely, the shape of *one surface* (or cross-section) of the block and that of the *base*, or the 'bed' (as one of our subjects expressed it) which the porcelain formed for it. Similarly, in relating ring F to D, the 'shape' fundaments do not include the squareness of F's cross-section nor the shape of D as viewed laterally, but are restricted to the shape of F's circumference and to that of the threaded part of D. In both cases the 'sizes' of the shape fundaments also function, but in less determinate fashion than would have been the case had (say) a number of different sized rings been provided.

Concerning 'number', as a character this did not appear to function in the same essential way as 'shape', but contingently, owing to there being in the porcelain test a duplication of parts. The educed relation (identity) between parts of the same number did not lead immediately to insight into their mechanical relation, but served to direct attention to the more essential characters of 'shape' and 'function'.

Regarding 'function', its apprehension was a more complex process than that of apprehending shape, since it was effected by associating with the apprehended shapes a reproduced knowledge of the purpose served by such shaped objects. In the present tests, this was restricted to such knowledge concerning the general purpose of screws and springs as all subjects possess. As fundaments, such 'functional' characters functioned more clearly in the process of finding correlates than in that of finding relations, with which we are at present concerned. Nevertheless, some eduction of relations of the kind we have called 'functional' occurred, as between the screw and the hole into which it fitted. This was usually closely associated with the above-mentioned eduction of relations between their shapes and sizes.

(ii) *The relations.* Of the various relations which *might* have been educed, those which actually functioned were principally those of 'similarity', of 'identity' and of the kind we have called 'functional'— 'similarity', when the fundaments which actually functioned (e.g. the elementary shape characters, such as the shape of one surface) were not clearly differentiated from other closely associated characters (e.g. the shape of the complex whole); 'identity', when the fundaments so related were clearly differentiated. Relations of 'functionality' have already been described: they may be defined as those which function when one object is known to be the functional counterpart of the other. The fundaments between which such functional relations mediate are themselves frequently 'functional' in character, but not necessarily so—as when it is known, from the shape of the hole in L and of the flange on I, without any prior reference to their separate functions, that the two pieces will hold together in the way required. Many examples of the eduction of all these kinds of relation have already been given in our general description of this work. There we noticed that many of the simpler relations came readily to view in the first step, and formed the starting point for the manipulative work which, in turn, provided the experience whence were educed the more complex ones.

(*d*) *Functional disintegration of shape.* It is instructive to compare the eduction of relations between shapes with the apprehension of shape itself. We have seen that the latter involves the apprehension, *as a unitary whole*, of certain more elementary characters, together with their space relations, and that both characters and relations are integrated into a single complex shape by the single act of apprehension. Where, as is usual, only certain of the more elementary characters of the shape function as fundaments in the eductive process, it is evident that the converse must occur—the complex shape will be disintegrated into its more elementary constituents. In so far as these latter, as we have shown, frequently lack clear differentiation from one another when functioning in the eductive process, the disintegration seems best described as a functional one.

Although these observations seem to us fundamental to any theory of shape perception, space forbids their further elaboration. Their practical import seems to lie in two suggestions to which they point, namely, (i) that persons who find it difficult to apprehend complex shapes might also find it difficult to disintegrate them, and (ii) that special training in assembling work might profitably include practice in such integrating and disintegrating operations.

(*e*) *Eduction of correlates.* (i) *Correlative characters.* We have seen that many of the 'characters' involved in these processes are known by simple apprehension. Sometimes, however, there intervenes an eductive process of the kind known as correlate eduction. This occurs when the observing of the character of some part leads to a definite search after another part, having some preconceived character. This preconceived character is the educed correlate. For example, a hole is observed of a certain size and shape which leads to a looking for a screw to fit it. Here the given fundament is the size and shape of the hole, and the given relation that of 'similarity', whence is educed the characters (shape and size) which the object to fit the hole must have. By reproductive association it is at once known that such characters inhere in a screw. Such educed characters may, of course, possess varying degrees of generality and obscurity, which only become particularized and clear when the object having these characters is discovered. An example of great generality in the educed character was the looking for projections on to which the grooves on *B* might set; and one of both generality and obscurity, in the looking for 'something which would hold the spring and allow it to work'.

(ii) *Correlative space relations.* We have yet to consider one further relation, that of space between the parts to be assembled. It was, of course, knowledge of how the various parts were related in space that formed the ultimate goal of all other mental activity—to know it was to know how to assemble the object. To make clear the process involved in attaining this knowledge, consider the simple case of discovering that block *L* fits into the porcelain 'bed'. The steps in the process are (i) noting certain characters of the shapes of these two pieces, (ii) noting the similarity between these, and (iii) noting the relative spatial positions into which these may be placed (e.g. the block in its bed) on account of this relationship. Clearly (iii) is educed as a correlate where (ii) is the initially given fundament, and the relation known as that of 'evidence' is the mediating relation. The evidence that the parts *may* occupy the proposed positions is derived from previous knowledge as to how things of given shape, size, or function may be fitted together. That they actually *do* occupy these positions is not, as a rule, immediately evident from previous knowledge alone, but from general experience, conjoined with such indications as are given by the work which has already been done on the test itself.

In the foregoing example, the given fundament was the similarity between two shape elements. But any other of the relations we have been discussing might have functioned equally well. Usually, the fundament will be a complex of as many of these 'indicating' relations as may have been cognized. In general, then, the ultimate process whereby the relative positions of the various parts in the assembled object are known is that of the eduction of correlates in which the given fundament is any or all of the relations we have described above, and the given relation is that of 'evidence'.

(iii) *Comparison with apprehension of shape.* An interesting comparison may be made between this process of placing the parts into correct spatial relationships and that of apprehending shape. When the object is completed it has a complex shape, of which the shapes of its parts are the more elementary constituents. The space relations between these parts correspond to those between what we have called the more elementary spatial characters of a shape. We have seen that the knowing of the space relations between its parts is a condition for knowing the shape itself. Similarly, to be able to assemble the object (at least mentally) is to know the space relations between its parts.

There are, however, three ways in which the task of mentally constructing the object differs from that of apprehending shape. First, in the former case the space relations have to be constructed or invented, whereas in the latter they are given with the characters themselves, and merely await cognition. It is true that this invention of relations is governed by the conditions of the problem—as is all invention—and that in the present tests the relations to be invented were strictly determined by the shapes of the parts and the object to be made from them. Nevertheless, the inventing is a prior condition to knowing whether the invention is satisfactory.

The second difference is seen in the fact that the further process of apprehending the elementary characters together with their relation, essential to shape apprehension, is not necessary to object construction. The latter may stop short at the stage of 'knowing all about the shape', to which we have previously referred. Indeed, to *apprehend* the shape of even our relatively simple objects with clearness of detail would be beyond the power of many subjects who yet succeeded in assembling their parts.

Although not essential, it is clearly helpful to be able to cognize the shape that would result from any proposed assemblage of parts, for by so doing one could more readily foresee the result, and could select mentally from a number of proposed alternatives the mode of assemblage that best suited the purpose; not to be able to do so, when assembling, may be compared to the position of a designer who can get little notion of what effect the elements he proposes in his design will have until he actually puts them in. This knowledge of what would result from any proposed mode of assemblage comes by way of correlate eduction, in which the shapes of the various parts, with their proposed relationships, form the given fundament, and the relation is that of 'constitution', whence is educed the shape so constituted. Herein lies the third difference between this and the apprehension of shape.

From what has been said, we should expect those who are poor at apprehending shapes and designs to be poor at the more complex task of inventing them. Observations on children confirm this view. Teachers of art, needlework and other forms of handicraft seem agreed that children even in the upper classes of elementary schools have the greatest difficulty in *creating* any but simple geometrical designs. At the same time, they can *appreciate* much more complex ones, for they choose ready-made designs, if further labour, such as embroidery, is to be spent on them, rather than use their own, which they regard as not worth while. This difference between creating and appreciating, between inventing and understanding, would seem to spring from the above described differences in mental processes.

A good example of the difficulty experienced by children in dealing with the relations involved in designing is shown in the efforts of a boy[1] aged 8, depicted in fig. 53. A simple design with daffodils and leaves,

[1] My son Claude.

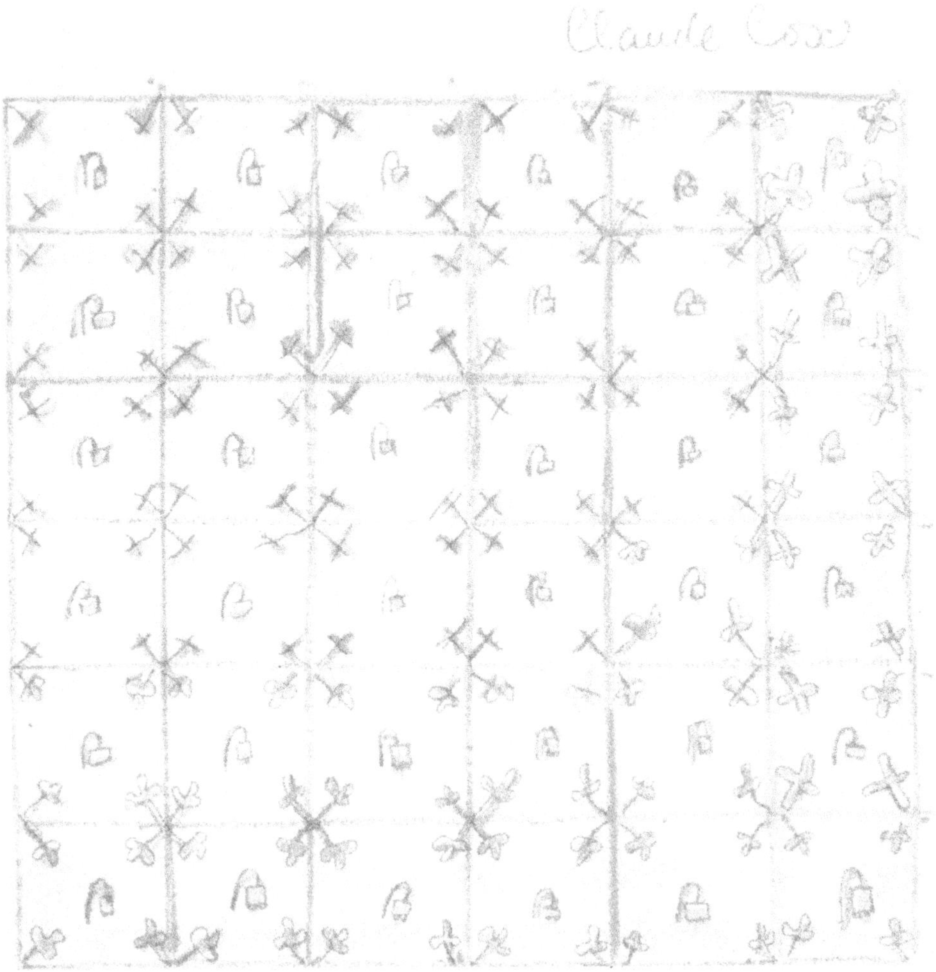

Fig. 53. Design by a boy aged eight years

in which all these objects were interwoven and connected together, was first drawn while the child looked on. He was then asked to make up a design for himself, with the result shown.

(*f*) *Reproductive processes*. The tests were carried out, of course, on a general background of everyday knowledge. The conditions under which this reproduced knowledge became associated with that arrived at by the above-described eductive processes have already been referred to in describing the latter. Therefore we mention them here merely for the sake of completeness.

As we have seen, reproduced knowledge was confined generally to (i) knowledge of the general functions carried out by screws and springs, (ii) knowledge of the general conditions regulating the relations in space which one thing can bear to another (such as, that two things cannot occupy the same space simultaneously, that a thing cannot pass through a hole smaller than itself, and that areas of similar size and shape will coincide), (iii) knowledge of the general shape of a lamp-holder, and (iv) knowledge that *all* the parts must be so fitted together as to make a complete whole in which all are functionally related.

(*g*) *'Functional' selection*. Our description would be seriously lacking if we omitted one further remark—not on a mental process but on a general feature of the activity throughout, namely its purposive character. The processes which we have examined were not manifested as random elements in an assortment of other processes; they were governed by an aim. This aim did not determine the precise order in which the processes occurred. The order depended partly upon the subject's ability and knowledge, and partly upon chance. But the aim determined the *general character* of the fundaments and relations. Had our subject been set a different task with the same pieces, such as to draw or to paint them, quite other characters and relations would have functioned. The interesting point about such selective apprehension and eduction is that, although they are certainly purposive in the sense that they are governed by the purpose in view, the selection itself is not made, as it were, *on purpose*—there is no conscious selection of certain characters and rejection of others, no conscious decision as to the sort of relation one shall choose, or try to see, between the characters. One simply 'sees' the kind relevant to the purpose in view. We, therefore, suggest the term 'functional selection' for this general characteristic of all purposive cognitive activity.

CHAPTER XV

SUBJECTIVE ANALYSIS OF 'ROUTINE' ASSEMBLING

A. GENERAL DESCRIPTION OF THE MENTAL ACTIVITY

1. Two kinds of activity.

It will be remembered that in routine operations the task is limited to the manual work involved in assembling the material, and that the activity referred to in the last chapter as 'Activity II' is directed to the same end. We have now to consider the mental activity involved in this manual work, confining attention, for the present, to its cognitive (or thinking) aspect.[1]

This cognitive activity can be sharply divided into two kinds, according to the sort of knowledge it yields. The first kind, which we shall call 'Activity A', leads, when successful, to knowledge of the movements to be imparted to the material; the second kind, 'Activity B', is directed towards knowing how best to impart these movements. The distinction may be made clear by some typical examples.

(a) *Activity A—leading to knowledge of the objective spatial characters of the movements to be imparted to the material.* Let us first consider the relatively simple operation of assembling screws. To do this, the small screw[2] K is picked up in the fingers of the right hand (in right-handed subjects), and the block L in the fingers of the left hand. The two are brought together so that the tip of the screw covers the entrance to the hole in the block, and the length of the screw is at right angles to the surface in which the hole occurs. The screw is then pushed forward into the hole until a resistance to further movement is felt, whereupon it is given a sharp turn. If the screw is felt to 'bite', the operation is finished. If not first pushed 'home' (i.e. until the resistance is felt), the screw will not bite; if it is home but not 'straight' (i.e. at right angles to the surface of the block) at the moment it is turned, it will jam. It is evident that such faults will frequently occur unless the

---

[1] The bodily (neuro-muscular) aspect is, of course, outside the scope of this psychological investigation.

[2] The parts referred to in this chapter will be found in fig. 1 (p. 31).

subject is clear about these necessary characters of the screw's movement, viz. the forward motion with screw 'straight', followed by a turn at the right signal.

Further examples occur plentifully in the more complex material. Thus, in the porcelain operation, the most difficult part—the assemblage of the screw *H*—was made very much easier by realizing that (i) the pin *I* should be allowed to pass as far as possible through the hole in the block *L* (into which it fits), (ii) the spring *G* should be pushed to the bottom of the pin (not held up on the flange or on the block), and (iii) the screw *H* should be pushed downwards (against the upward force of the spring), until it is felt to be 'home' (in the hole of *L*) before being turned, and must be kept 'straight' (with this hole) as it is turned.

Knowledge of a similar kind is called for in the assembling of 'wedges'. Here the operation is facilitated if, as the wedges are inserted, their coincident surfaces are prevented from slipping. In assembling the 'container', the porcelain *M* must move into *D* as far as possible, so that, when *C* is placed over the rim of *M*, it will be close enough to *D* to allow the ring *E* to reach from *D* to *C* (to which it must be screwed).

This knowledge of the shape of the movement, and of its spatial relations to certain other parts of the material, decides the subject on the sort of movement he *intends* to impart. It is clearly distinguishable from the ability to carry out this intention, and from that which results from the Activity I of our last chapter. Whereas the latter consists in knowing the positions of the parts when assembled (as for example where a certain screw goes), the former consists in knowing how the parts must move in order to reach these positions (e.g. the positions in which the screw must be held to get it into place). It resembles Activity I, seeing that it could conceivably be acquired in complete independence of the assembling operation itself—by a careful study of the parts, with the aid of sectional diagrams, or by verbal communication.

In this respect, it differs radically from another way in which these self-same movements of material must be known if they are to be imparted skilfully, viz. in terms of the subjective experience undergone while actually imparting them—a matter to be considered later as part of Activity B. At the same time, these two ways of knowing are acquired in close dependence on one another. While the objective character which the movement is thought to require guides the sub-

14-2

jective act, the ensuing subjective experience often serves to make clearer the objective spatial characters of the movement. Thus, from its visual appearance, the screw may be judged to require a certain amount of turn to make it 'bite'; but this quantitative character of the screw's movement is known much more accurately after one has done the actual turning. In converse manner, the known spatial characters may clarify knowledge of the correlative subjective experience, e.g. seeing that the screw is turning 'straight' enables one to know the subjective experience associated with this kind of movement.

(b) *Activity B—leading to knowledge concerning the way to bring about the requisite movements.* The first kind of activity concerns knowledge of what the material must do. The second type concerns how to make the material do it. More precisely, under Activity B are classified the various mental operations involved in so employing one's fingers and tools that movements having the necessary characters are imparted to the material.

As a simple illustration, we may revert to the operation of inserting the screw in the block. Even when the spatial characters of the movement which the screw must undergo are known, the subject will often fail to get the screw in successfully. Although he knows that the screw must first be pushed 'home' and 'straight', he may (i) turn it before it has reached this position, whereupon it falls out on being released (or jams); or (ii) fail to keep the screw 'straight' as he turns it, with similar results as before; or (iii) find that he is holding the screw in such a way that his finger-tips come in contact with the block as he turns the screw, thus making the necessary movement awkward or impossible.

In (i), he fails to wait for the peculiar feel of the pressure against the finger-tips which announces that the screw is 'home'. In (ii), failure may be due to either of *two* sources; he may not be very clear about the direction and magnitude of the forces needed to turn the screw and at the same time keep it straight; or, knowing this, he may not succeed in placing and moving his fingers in just the way needed to impart forces of this requisite character. In (iii), his present failure (or handicap) arises from some earlier circumstance, namely, the picking up of the screw badly in the first instance.

2. SUBDIVISIONS OF ACTIVITY B.

These four sources of failure illustrate four kinds of mental activity into which that broadly designated Activity B may be divided. The basis of division is, as before, the knowledge which results from the activity. These activities are not, of course, manifested independently. The success of one will frequently depend upon the success of the other—just as the course of Activity II (in the mechanical assembling operations) was seen to modify that of Activity I.[1]

Before attempting to analyse the activities themselves it will be helpful to look at some further examples, with a view to indicating more clearly the nature of the knowledge with which each is concerned.

(*a*) *Knowledge of 'signals'*. The first kind may be described as knowing when to initiate a certain kind of movement. This, in turn, depends on knowing the appropriate signal for its initiation. Thus, in the above example, the turning movement of the screw is the movement to be initiated; the pressure of the finger-tips is the chief (though not the sole) signal for its initiation.

Similar cases are seen in the screwing of *A* and of *E* on to *C*, and of *F* on to *D*. In each case the thread on the piece to be assembled must be adjusted 'straight' with that on to which it is to be screwed, before the screwing motion is imparted. It is, therefore, essential to know—by what we have called the 'signals'—when this adjustment has been effected, so that the movements involved in adjusting one to the other may give place to those of screwing up.

A more difficult 'signal' to interpret is that which informs the subject that the thread of screw *H* is in correct adjustment with the hole in *L*, into which it is to be screwed. The difficulty is increased (i) by the distraction imposed by two other difficult operations which must be carried out at the same time—(*a*) the downward thrust on the screw (against the pressure of the spring) by the driver in the right hand, and (*b*) the holding of the block in position on the porcelain (against the resulting downward thrust on it) by skilful handling with the left; and (ii) by the interpolation of a tool (the screwdriver) between the occurrence to be 'signalled' and the kinaesthetic sensations in the fingers upon which its interpretation depends.

We shall refer to this operation of bringing the pieces into correct spatial relation in preparation for the next movement as one of 'adjustment'. The underlying cognitive processes (considered later) clearly divide into (i) those concerned with bringing the pieces into adjustment, and (ii) those which convey the 'signal' that the adjust-

---

[1] For example, unless the screw is inserted 'straight' the appropriate 'signal' for turning the screw will not be receivable.

ment has been effected. It is the latter that are referred to in the present section as underlying the *interpretation* of the 'signal'. The former fall among the processes which have yet to be considered.

So far, we have mentioned only those 'signals' which indicate that an adjustment of one part to another has been *correctly* effected.

For completeness they must be extended to include *any* indication that some change must be made in the magnitude or duration of the forces that are being directed on to the material. Such will occur when movements go wrong and call for readjustments—the signal, for example, that the screw has gone 'crooked', or has not 'bitten'. But, whereas these will be of less frequent occurrence as the subject becomes more skilful, and will vary from trial to trial according to the errors made, the 'terminal' signals will remain throughout as special objectives, or sign-posts, marking the route which the material must take.

We ought also to include all those signs that give continuous indication as to what is happening between the occurrences of the above 'signals'—for example, that the screw is being turned with a certain speed, and that the block L is being pressed against the porcelain with an appropriate amount of force and in the right direction. These do not seem to differ in essential psychological character from the 'adjustment' class, but are distinguishable in that the latter indicate a turning point necessitating a change in the mode of manipulating the material; these 'guiding' signs indicate that the movement is proceeding satisfactorily and may be continued (or repeated). They also differ in their claim on attention. The adjustment kind are special objects of attention to be actively sought after and regarded focally; whereas those concerned in guiding the movement enter marginally—the central object of attention at the time being the physical object moved.

(*b*) *Knowledge of the forces to be imparted to* (i) *the material*, (ii) *the body* (*fingers*). We have now to consider the case where the subject has correctly interpreted the signal and knows the sort of movement 'signalled', but fails to carry it out.[1] The cognitive work necessary to avert such failure divides into two parts: (i) that concerned with objective forces and movements, and (ii) that concerned with the subjective experience associated with these forces and movements. These will form the respective topics of our present and next subsections.

To return to the case where the subject, having correctly received

[1] I.e. fails to impart to the material a movement having the right spatial characters (as cognized by Activity A).

the signal to turn the screw and knowing that it should be kept 'straight', fails to keep it 'straight' as he turns it. Such failure *may* result from not knowing that as the turning movement is made the pressures of the thumb and finger on the screw-head must be of equal magnitude and act in opposite directions in a plane at right angles to the axis around which the screw rotates.[1]

A more difficult problem of the same kind was encountered in the 'porcelain' operation. Here the block L and porcelain M had to be held together between the thumb and forefinger of the left hand in such a way that the downward pressure exerted on the block as the screw was screwed in (by the screwdriver in the right hand) was counteracted by an appropriate thrust from the finger to keep the block in position. Almost invariably this thrust was at first exerted in a direction (roughly upward) immediately opposed to that of the screw, whereupon the block tended to move outwards. To meet this difficulty, the finger would be transferred to the end of the block to exert an inward pressure; whereupon, the upward pressure being reduced, the block would move downwards. Finally (usually after other attempts at holding and thrusting the block in various ways), the finger would move to the bottom of the block and exert a thrust intermediate in direction to these 'upward' and 'inward' thrusts—one that would keep it both 'up' and 'in'.

It is clear that wherever a force is to be applied to the material—whether to keep a part in position or to bring about a desired movement—its characters, such as its 'magnitude', 'direction', 'duration', 'rate', and 'point of application', must be known.[2] Since these determine the mechanical effects, they may be appropriately termed 'mechanical' characters.

In similar fashion, the efforts which activate the various parts of the body will vary in 'mechanical' character according to the part activated, the amount of effort made, the rate at which it is made, the position of the part, etc.

Thus, the mechanical character of the effort needed to bend the finger differs from that needed to stretch it; that which produces a sudden bend differs from that required to produce a slow one. These

---

[1] In the case of this simple turning movement, most subjects will have already acquired such knowledge in the course of ordinary experience, although they may not be able to analyse it mechanically.

[2] With varying degrees of clearness dependent on the accuracy required in the force.

characters of the efforts which operate the fingers are not the same as those of the forces which the fingers impart to the material.[1] But the former determine the latter and must therefore be known. The disposition of the whole body in general, and of the hand and fingers in particular, will be decided by the subject according to the mechanical characters with which he wishes to endow the forces acting on the material, and to those of the efforts by which he intends to operate his fingers in bringing these forces about. To change the hand from an awkward, fatiguing position to a more comfortable one is frequently to alter the character of the effort, the resultant force in the material remaining the same.

One of the factors in skilful movement is clear awareness of the characters of the effort needed. The absence of this is seen in the difficulty experienced in making the fingers move as one wishes during the early attempts at a new manual operation. The requisite characters may be known with varying degrees of precision. Thus, in the assembling operations, the characters of the efforts involved in such well-known movements as picking up the material, bringing the parts together, grasping the handle of the driver, and turning the screws, were known with a high degree of precision from the first, although, even here, knowledge became more precise in the course of practice.[2] In the entirely new operation of fixing the block to the porcelain the characters of the needed efforts were largely unknown at first.

As with physical forces, the mechanical characters of these subjective efforts are known (and discovered) by their effects, i.e. by the way the finger (or other part) is observed to move when the effort is made. Thus, in turning the screw, the particular kind of effort made to move the finger and thumb in the way thought necessary to turn the screw may be observed to result in a bending of the finger which pulls the screw crooked. On observing this bending of the finger, an attempt may be made to change the character of the effort in such a way that no bending occurs when the twisting movement is made. In so doing, great assistance is derived from certain characters which, unlike 'mechanical' characters, these bodily efforts do not share with the

---

[1] Thus, the forces operating on the hand which holds and turns the screwdriver are very different, 'mechanically', from the resultant forces which turn the screw.

[2] For example, the precise distribution and amount of effort needed (and no more) to grasp the driver firmly; the precise amount of movement to give the fingers when twisting the screw (by hand); the precise distance through which the hand must move to reach the material on the bench.

physical forces, namely, their 'subjective' characters, which we shall now consider.

Before turning to these, it may, however, be remarked that the mechanical effects are frequently thought of as resulting from the *movement* of the finger or tool (when movement occurs), rather than from the force exerted when it moves. In this sense, the movements may be thought of as having 'mechanical' characters.

(*c*) *Knowledge of the subjective characters of the appropriate efforts and movements of the body (fingers).* So far as their 'mechanical' characters are concerned, the subjective efforts and the bodily parts which they move stand in the same relation to mind as do objective forces and things. If no other source of knowledge were open to us, we should know our fingers merely as objective mechanical tools, to be used this way or that according to their mechanical possibilities. Thus limited, we should be for ever compelled to watch our fingers to see what they were doing. Like a bad workman with his tools, we should be in constant danger of damaging them; and—largely for the same reason— we should have no direct information as to how they were getting on in the task we had set them. We should not know, for example, whether the upward thrust of the left forefinger was far greater than was needed (to keep the block in position against the downward thrust of the right hand transmitted through the screwdriver), and so was unduly fatiguing the muscles; whether, on the contrary, the block would be pushed aside unless the thrust thereon were increased; whether the gradual increase in the downward thrust (arising from the compression of the spring) was being met by a corresponding increase in the upward thrust of the left forefinger just sufficient to keep the block in position. We should have no clear 'signals'; for the knowledge 'signalled' through the 'motor' sense is far more exact here than that derived from vision, and the effects they indicate usually originate in parts of the material hidden from view. We should, in short, be in a similar state of knowledge regarding the disposal of our efforts as is the engineer regarding the arrangement of the forces in his material, and we should equally need pressure gauges and a science of mechanics in order to use our fingers efficiently.

Happily, this needful knowledge is provided without resort to any such clumsy and indirect method. It is provided immediately in the subjective experience which accompanies the disposal of our efforts. There is no need to measure and calculate, as with physical forces—for the simple reason that we can 'feel' what our fingers are doing. More exactly, each particular kind of effort has a distinctive subjective character, which distinguishes it from another. Thus, the sort of effort required to close the hand is 'felt' (or more correctly 'cognized') to be different from that required to open it. The effort needed to effect a light touch differs again from that required to execute a firm pressure; and that required to move any bodily part quickly from that required to move the same part slowly. These characters convey knowledge of the magnitude of the effort and of its manner of distribution in the bodily parts (mainly the fingers), through which it is conveyed to the material.

These subjective characters (of the efforts) are distinguishable from another class, viz. those belonging to the movements of the body which result from the efforts. Each movement (or combination of movements) has its distinctive subjective character which enables one to determine how the part (or parts) in question is moving. The difference between the two is observable on comparing the experience of moving (say) a finger with that of having the same finger moved in the same way by someone else. In the former case, characters of both effort and movement are to be apprehended; in the latter, the characters of effort are absent.

(*d*) *Knowledge anticipating subsequent finger movements.* I consider, finally, the case where the subject is obstructed in his movements by his manner of holding the material. The remedy lies in foreseeing the circumstance, and in so modifying one's method of handling that the awkward position is avoided. In example (iii) of p. 212, this was done by picking up the screw with its end well projecting beyond the finger-tips. Such foresight depends on realizing, before the hands are placed in position, (i) the sort of movement required of them when in position, and (ii) the relation in space between (*a*) the positions through which the fingers must pass to execute the movement and (*b*) the positions which the material (or other parts of the hand) will occupy while the movement is in progress.

B. THE COGNITIVE PROCESSES

1. CONSTITUTING ACTIVITY A.

We have now reviewed the chief kinds of knowledge called for in the routine operations, and it remains to examine the cognitive processes upon whose successful functioning the acquirement of this knowledge depends.

The Activity A processes, it will be remembered, bring knowledge about the positions and the movements to be imparted to the parts of the material during the assembling operation—such as knowledge of the distance the screw should enter the hole before being turned, of the amount of turning necessary before the screw 'bites', of the distance the spring must enter the pin before putting on the screw, of the necessity of keeping parts *C* and *D* close together while assembling the ring *E*. These we have called the 'spatial' characters of the movements of the material.

The underlying processes fall into three main classes, namely, reproductive, eductive and apprehensive, as follows:

(*a*) *Reproduction of the general spatial characters of the movements required.* All subjects had carried out the 'mechanical' assembling operations before doing the 'routine' assembling; and all knew the function of such things as rings, springs and screws. Hence, all started the routine operation with a knowledge of the general direction which the movement of the part should take—that the screw should be turned clockwise, that the spring should be pushed through the hole into the pin, etc. Here, then, the process is one of simple reproduction (or recall). The recalled item is the direction to be imparted to the movement (in relation to other parts) and the reproducing process follows upon the simple apprehension of the shape of the part and the recognition of its function.

(*b*) *Eduction of the particular spatial characters of the movements required.* This general knowledge must be applied to the particular material. Hence, it is not enough to know (for example) that the screw 'turns' in the hole—the relation in space which this particular screw must bear to this particular hole while being turned must be known, as also the amount of turn necessary to cause the screw to hold (or 'bite'); and, similarly, as regards the movement of other parts. To arrive at this particular knowledge, one must know (i) the relations in space between the hole and the surface of the block in which it occurs, and (ii) the relations in space which the screw must bear to the hole in order to enter it. These make it possible to know (iii) the relations which the screw must bear to the block while turning, i.e. the particular character of the screw's movement.[1] In (i) the process consists in educing the relation in space between certain characters of the

[1] Guidance in effecting this movement was provided by the relation between screw and block rather than between screw and hole.

cylindrical space occupied by the hole—especially, its longitudinal axis, and certain characters of the space occupied by the block—in particular, the surface in which the hole enters. (ii) in the present operations is usually reproduced from previous experience. When the particular knowledge is lacking, it may be educed as a correlate from the observed shapes of the objects ('screw' and 'hole') and from the known way in which things must be related in space in order to re-act mechanically with each other. If this becomes too difficult, resort must be made to actual trial after the manner described in (*c*) below. The knowledge (iii) is gained by the process of correlate eduction, in which not only the mediating relations, but also the fundaments, are space relations. Thus, the space relation between the hole and the block is known from (i) and serves as the given fundament; the screw is known from (ii) to be *similarly* related—which supplies the given relation; hence is educed the correlative position of the screw in relation to the block. This correlative position 'at right angles to the surface of the block' thus becomes known as one of the characters that must be given to the screw's movement.

In a similar way, the relative positions in which *C*, *D* and *E* must be held, in order to 'start the thread' when *E* is turned, may be educed from the position of the threads on *C* and *D* and from the known relation which the thread on *E* must bear, in space, to these.

(*c*) *Apprehension of the characters—mainly quantitative—of the movements observed.* The characters so far considered are known from the observed shapes and sizes of the various parts. They provide the basis of knowledge upon which one proceeds to act. On attempting to impart the movements thus thought to be necessary, further knowledge of the way in which the pieces should be moved may come to light by observing the response which the material actually makes. This may arise in two ways: (i) When the result is unsuccessful, attention may be drawn to certain characters of the shapes of the parts (such as the projections on *C*) which had been formerly overlooked and which necessitate a change in the characters that the movement was formerly thought to require. Here the mental processes are the same as described above in (*b*), the only difference between the two situations being the conditions under which the relevant items of experience become evoked. (ii) When the movement is successful, certain characters, mainly quantitative, which were previously known only in an approximate way, if at all, may be directly observed. The distance through which the screw must be turned to make it hold, the number of turns needed to complete the assembly of *F* and of *E*, and the distance into the hole in the porcelain through which *H* must be pushed (by the driver) in order to reach the block into which it fixes, are examples of these quantitative characters.

Where the positions and movements of the material are associated with definite correlative positions of the fingers, their characters may be apprehended through both the visual and the motor senses. Thus, the amount of turning to be given to the screw to make it 'bite' is known not only by the distance through which the finger is seen to move in relation to the thumb, but also (and probably more accurately) by the amount of turning movement the fingers are 'felt' to undergo.

2. CONSTITUTING ACTIVITY B.

The mental processes just considered lead to insight into the nature (spatial characters) of the movements which the material must undergo during the process of assembling. To cognize these characters clearly is of course an essential step towards effecting a skilful assembly: conversely, the assembling activity itself frequently provides the circumstance for making clearer these spatial characters (through the motor sense, as observed above). Beyond thus providing the manual activity with its aim, viz. to impart movements of the cognized character, the processes of Activity A bring no knowledge as to how the necessary manual activity is to be carried out. This knowledge, we have seen, divides into four broad classes which we will now proceed to examine more closely.

(*a*) *Cognizing 'signals'.* Consider the case of cognizing that the screw *H* is 'home' in the hole and 'straight' with the hole—hence ready for the turn. The necessary knowledge is derived from both visual and motor sources. When the screw is *seen* to be 'straight' (at right angles with the block surface) and to resist any further forward movement, it is judged to be ready to turn. In other words, the relation in space between the screw and the block is recognized as having the two characters which it was known to require in the light of Activity A.

Thus far the process is that of simple eduction and identification of the space relation between the two parts ('screw' and 'block') of the visual percept. But accompanying the seen cessation of the screw's forward movement is the felt backward pressure on the finger-tips which hold the screw; and accompanying the seen 'straightness' are the positions in space in which the screw and the block are 'felt' to be held. The space relation between these felt positions may be educed. The turning movement to be given is 'signalled', as before, when this relation has been cognized as 'straight with each other'. In cognizing the 'straightness', vision seems to be more relied on at first; but as practice proceeds and the positions of the pieces become 'felt' with greater clearness and accuracy, the task of presenting the experience (on which the apprehensive and eductive processes work) falls largely on the 'motor' sense. The 'home' position seemed cognized through the 'motor' sense (mainly that of light pressure) from the beginning. Throughout, however, knowledge derived from the one source confirmed that derived from the other, although, with the present writer, the final word rested with the 'motor' sense—it was not enough for the screw to 'look' straight with the hole (although this was necessary), it had also to 'feel' straight.

Cognizing the 'felt' position of the pieces is not, of course, an elementary process. How, it may be asked, does one come to know the positions of the screw and block without looking at them? The existence of such knowledge is evidenced by the ability to bring the block and screw into correct relative positions with the eyes shut. The cognitive processes appear to be as follows: (i) the positions in space of the points of contact of the screw-head with the finger-tips are known from the positions of the touch stimuli on the fingers (given as a character of the touch sensations) and the position in space of the fingers (given as a complex character of the kinaesthetic sensations aroused in bringing and maintaining the fingers in this position); (ii) the shape of the whole screw is known already (by previous visual or tactual exploration); (iii) the part of the screw in contact with the fingers is recognized from the educed spatial relations between the points of contact and the known shape of that part—with the help of further tactual exploration bringing more points of contact, if necessary; (iv) the position in space of this part of the screw (the 'head') is educed as a correlate from the known positions of its points of contact with the fingers (as the fundament), which are given in immediate sensory experience as described in (i) above, and from the known space relation which this part bears to these points of contact; (v) the position in space of the remainder of the screw (and hence the screw as a whole) is similarly educed from this (now) known position of its part and from the space relation (known as a character of its shape) which the remainder bears to this part. In similar fashion is educed the position of the block (held in the other hand). Hence may be educed (without looking) the space relation between the two positions.[1]

The motor sense assumes special importance in cognizing the position of screw H in the assemblage of porcelains; for the block into which this screw must be fitted is not visible, and the position of the screw in relation to the block (the 'signal') must be cognized *via* a screwdriver.

The cognitive processes are essentially of the same kind as in the above case where the screw is held in the hand. The position of the block is educed from the 'felt' position of the part which touches the finger engaged in pressing it against the porcelain part M and the space relation which this part is known (from the shape of the block) to bear to the remainder. The mental operation of cognizing the position of the screw is more complex, since this is derived from (i) the position of the screwdriver, and (ii) the character of the resistance at the end of the driver; but the processes are of the same kind. The first is educed[2] from the 'felt' position of the part held in the hand (as in the previous examples). The position of the screw is cognized as 'straight' in the hole, and 'home' (the 'signal' for the turn) when the space relation between the educed positions of driver and block is that known as 'straight', and the character of the resistance of the screw-head to the forward thrust of the driver is 'felt' to be 'firm and even, with no tendency to wobble'. This 'felt' character of the resistance is not, of course, a feeling in the true psychological sense. It is, itself, educed from changes in the characters of the pressures transmitted to the fingers which hold and thrust the block and the driver, and from their relation (known in a general way from everyday experience, and learnt more accurately in the present application during practice) to changes in the positions of the things held and thrust.

In all this, the work is greatly supplemented and confirmed by visual experience.[3] Thus, the driver is not only 'felt' to be 'straight', but is also 'seen' to be so; and the screw-head is seen to be 'level' with the end of the driver. But in the last determination that the ap-

---

[1] The operation here analysed can be readily introspected by trying to bring together, with eyes closed, the points of two pencils, held, between the finger tips, one in each hand.
[2] In the absence of vision.
[3] This does not apply to the block, for it is out of sight.

propriate conditions for successfully turning the screw are fulfilled, the cognitive work rooted in the motor experience seems the final arbiter. From the visual position of the screw-head one can only arrive at the approximate position of the screw's end, whereas the tactual and motor characters of the felt thrust on the driver and block convey the more important information as to how the end is behaving. This is an essential factor in reacting appropriately to that behaviour—a condition for imparting the requisite movement.

Before turning to this, it may be noted that, just as the happenings at these crucial points in the path of the material are 'signalled', so is 'signalled' what is happening all along the line. But between these 'signal' points the cognitive work plays a less essential part, either because (i) great accuracy of movement is not called for (as in placing *E* over *D*), or because (ii) the movements of the fingers are guided externally (as in screwing up after the screw has been adjusted to the thread). In these circumstances, the mind is not compelled to look so carefully, either through the eye or the hand. Yet these movements leave room for the development of skill; for screwing-up in a way which jags the thread and fatigues the fingers is hardly a 'skilled' performance. The kind of movements needed to avoid such faults are signalled by processes similar to those which we have seen to be necessary at the special 'danger' points.

(*b*) *Cognizing the characters of the required forces.* Having cognized the characters of the movement (or thrust) to be imparted and the signal for imparting the movement, it remains to impart this movement. We have seen that this involves knowing (i) the mechanical characters of the forces to be applied by the fingers, and (ii) the mode of so using the fingers that forces having these characters are imparted. Here we consider (i).

The processes underlying (i) are partly reproductive and partly eductive, according to the novelty of the experience. Thus, one knows from experience the 'direction' to be taken by the forces applied to the screw-head in order to turn it. On the basis of previous experience of the way things respond to forces, one first tries the kind of force that appears necessary. Where, as frequently happens, the material does not respond in the anticipated way, another force (or combination of forces) must be tried. Here the method is not entirely guesswork (or 'trial' and 'error'); one profits by the observed effects of the previous attempt. In this operation eductive processes again play an important rôle. Thus, on observing that neither an 'upward' nor an 'inward' force is of itself sufficient to keep the block L in position against the thrusts of the driver, one is not obliged to try another thrust at random. The direction of the required thrust can be educed (with more or less accuracy according to one's ability) as a correlate from the known directions of the two thrusts—already given—and from the relation which the new thrust must bear to these two (given in the knowledge that it must partake of something of the 'direction' of both). In similar fashion, the 'amount' of force to be imparted is learnt by the aid of eduction. When one presses too hard against the block, the fingers get tired. When they relax, the block shifts. Hence is educed (and exerted) an amount of pressure of intermediate magnitude. When this is still found to be unsatisfactory, it may form the starting point (fundament) for a further eductive effort. Where eduction is impossible, because the direction (or effect) of the unsuccessful force is not cognized clearly, one must resort to 'trial' and 'error'. A 'jab' with the screwdriver takes the place of a consciously directed turn. But only in the weakest subjects does the cognitive work fall to such a low level as that in pure 'trial and error'. Working on the observed effects of trials initially instigated in the light of general knowledge, the eductive processes lead, by more or less gradual steps, to a clearer insight into the 'mechanical' characters of the forces needed in the particular operation.

(*c*) *Cognizing the characters of bodily (finger) efforts and movements.* We have now to consider (ii) above. To use the fingers effectively one must know how to impart to the material (or tool), as rapidly as possible and with the minimum of fatigue, forces of the requisite 'mechanical' characters. Each particular effort (or system of efforts) made by the fingers is accompanied by a particular effect on the material (the force imparted), and by a particular subjective character derived from the sensations of touch, pressure and kinaesthesis (according to the kind of effort made). Each particular effort is thus known in two ways—objectively by its effects, subjectively by its accompanying complex of tactual and kinaesthetic sensations. The effort (including the ensuing finger movements, if any) is rightly directed when its effects on the material are such as to impart to it forces (including movements when these occur) of the right 'mechanical' character (as cognized by the processes described in (*b*)). The question here to be discussed is how these rightly directed movements come to be known.

The immediate effect of an effort is to impart a force or forces of a certain mechanical character to the finger or fingers; the secondary effect is to impart a force of a correlative (though not necessarily the same) character to the material. In habitual acts, the secondary effect has become so closely associated with the effort needed to bring it about that the primary effect is hardly thought of. Thus, in picking up the block, one attends to the secondary effect—the way one wishes to affect the block—leaving the very complex mechanical arrangement of the fingers and the amount of effort they exert to look after themselves. But, where the operation is a relatively new experience, the primary effect may call for considerable thought. If, for example, the block had been made of very delicate material and one wished to preserve its shape, one would need to consider carefully the disposition and pressure of the fingers and to watch closely their effect on the block.

Many of the efforts and movements in the assembling operations of the present research were of the habitual kind; as, for example, those involved in picking up the pieces and turning them into position. Here cognition seemed more concerned with determining what to do than with how to do it. In these cases it seemed sufficient to be clear about the characters of the movement (or force) to be imparted to the material, leaving the finger movements to look after themselves. But where these characters were of a novel kind, or were required in novel combination, as in turning the screw and at the same time keeping it straight with the hole, or inserting the wedges in *E* and at the same time keeping them together, the finger movements called for some consideration. The processes which contributed to the success of the operation under these circumstances may be classified as follows:

(i) *Cognizing the mechanical arrangement of the fingers.* Before imparting a force of given character to the material, the mode of arranging the fingers for this purpose must be known. Where this was not already known by experience the necessary knowledge had to be acquired. As a typical example, we may take the holding of the block *L* in position with the left hand while screwing up *H* with the right. The characters of the forces required in the material were—(i) a downward force on the porcelain, (ii) an equal and opposite force on the block, of sufficient magnitude to prevent the downward force of the screw while being screwed up from separating the block from the porcelain. The method adopted was to use the finger and thumb as a double lever. The finger would be placed under the block, and the thumb over the porcelain. At first these would be arranged as seemed best in the light of previous experience and knowledge of the general nature of the work which the fingers would be required to do. But, when the downward thrust on the block was actually experienced, the precise positions initially adopted were seldom found to be the most suitable; some rearrangement of finger and thumb was found necessary or advisable, in order better to meet and counter-act this downward thrust, and so to prevent the block from slipping either 'down' or 'out' from the porcelain. Such rearrangement consisted usually in moving the top of the finger nearer to the outer edge of the block so that its thrust could be directed not merely upward but also inward, thereby making use of the rim of the bed in which the block lies as anchorage against downward slipping, and devoting the energy thus saved to the inward component of the finger thrust to prevent outward slipping.

The problem here, then, is how best to use the tools provided (the fingers), in order to do the work required. As in determining the mechanical characters of the forces and movements in the material, so in determining the mechanical arrangement of the fingers, the processes are partly reproductive and partly eductive. In order to fulfil the general requirements of the situation, the usual arrangement 'finger on block, thumb on porcelain' is at once known as the customary method of holding two things together. Yet, in order to get the fingers into the best position, some further mental work involving the eduction of relations and of correlates is necessary. The direction in which the slipping of the block is observed to occur, as held initially, is apprehended as a character of the force acting on the block, and similarly as regards the direction in which the block was felt to push against the finger; these supply the given (complex) fundament. The relation in space which the direction of the required force must take in order to oppose successfully these two forces is known approximately from ordinary experience and supplies the needed relation. Hence is educed the direction in space which the new force must take. The new knowledge thus far secured relates to the nature of the force to be applied to the material. But it now remains to move the thumb and finger into a position whence a force of this character can be best applied. Here, again, given sufficient insight, the process is one of eduction, the educed correlate being such a position of finger and thumb as will enable a force of the required direction to be imparted to the material. The relations in space which the fingers must bear to one another and to the material held, in order to impart to it a particular force (or movement), supply the relation; the direction of the required force is the given fundament; whence may be educed the position on the block and porcelain into which the fingers must be moved to impart the needed force.

Such eductive work presupposes knowledge of the way in which the fingers must be arranged in relation to the material (i.e. the given relation), in order to exercise the required force. When this is absent, or the eductive ability weak, resort must be had to 'trial and error'. Even so, the digital arrangement adopted seems never wholly a guess; there seems always some eductive guidance, however dimly the fundaments and relations may be cognized. The difference between mere guessing and clear eduction appeared on observing the movements of a child of six. Her persistent efforts to attach the block to the porcelain invariably failed, largely because in her various attempts to keep the block from shifting while turning the screw she never hit upon the right position for the finger and thumb; and she was unable to educe this position, either through (i) inability to apprehend clearly the character of the thrust required on the block to parry that of the screw (the 'fundament'), or (ii) not knowing the space relation which her fingers must bear to the material in order to execute this thrust, or (iii) weakness in educing the correlative position to be taken up by her fingers.

(ii) *Cognizing the mode of activating the fingers.* After having arranged the fingers in correct spatial relation to the material, they must be activated in such a way as to impart forces having the requisite characters (as cognized by the processes described in (*b*) above). The relevant cognitive activity is intimately associated with the above described manner of arranging the fingers, since this arrangement is chosen not merely with regard to the forces to be applied to the material, but also in view of the kind of efforts[1] to be made (mainly) by the fingers when in position, i.e. their mode of activation. The mechanical arrangement, together with the subsequent mode of activation, constitute the subject's 'method'. To produce a given effect in the material there was usually some choice of method. But, when once the mechanical arrangement of the fingers had been adopted, there remained little choice as to their subsequent mode of activation.

[1] I.e. with respect to the characters of these efforts as described in (b) of Section A, p. 214.

The choice of method, within the limits imposed by the task, was largely determined by the ease with which the 'activation' part could be carried out. This itself was dependent on such inter-related factors as the flexibility of the joints, the habitual movements of the individual, and the sizes and shapes of the fingers. For example, in the porcelain operation, some chose to hold the block and porcelain together by placing the thumb on the former and the first two fingers on the latter: others preferred to reverse this position. The former method involved an awkward turn of the wrist but provided a stronger 'tool' —the thumb—where the greater force was needed.

Although the manner in which it is *intended* to activate the fingers is known when their mechanical arrangement is decided on, and partly determines this arrangement, it frequently happens that, like the arrangement itself, it is only known in a general way, which necessitates further cognitive work before the precise character of the necessary thrusts and movements of the fingers becomes clear. As an example, we may consider the case of turning the screw K and at the same time keeping it 'straight' with the hole. In this the *general* character of the movements needed of the fingers in order to impart the 'turning' was usually well known by long experience and was simply re-called; and similarly, as regards holding the screw in the 'straight' position. The new element consisted in learning to recognize the subjective characters (the 'feel') of the precise finger movements required and combining these in a single movement. This operation involves:

(i) Keeping before the mind a clear idea of the spatial characters[1] to be imparted to the movement of the screw while the activation of the fingers is in progress.

(ii) Educing the relative position of the screw and the block while the fingers are engaged in turning—by the same processes (visual and motor) as underlie the cognizing of 'signals' and are described in 2 (*a*) of the present section.

(iii) When the screw is cognized, in (ii) above, as 'not-straight', reacting by the necessary finger movement to replace it in the 'straight' position.

(iv) Clearly apprehending the complex subjective character of the whole finger movement when it is observed to be proceeding satisfactorily.

[1] As cognized by the processes described as Activity A.

(v) Associating this subjective character with the observed effect—'screw turning straight'.[1]

(vi) Recalling this character when it is desired to repeat the movement.

The processes involved in (iii) are similar to those involved in arranging the fingers prior to initiating their movements. The relation between the observed 'not-straight' position and the known 'straight' position is first educed. This determines the 'direction' of the movement to be imparted to the screw in order that it may regain the 'straight' position. Hence, the finger movement needed to produce this effect may be (i) recalled by previous association, or (ii) educed from the known relation in space which this finger movement must bear to the screw's movement, or (iii) arrived at by partial 'trial' where this relation is not clearly known.

The new character referred to in (iv) is composed of the more elementary and already known subjective characters associated with (i) the 'straight' position of the screw, and (ii) the turning position, together with the relation between them. These apprehended together yield knowledge—the 'felt' shape—of the new movement, in a fashion analogous to that involved in apprehending a new visual shape.[2]

The processes (v) and (vi) are memory processes, whereby, in the course of successive cognitive efforts, the newly apprehended subjective character of the requisite finger movement becomes so identified with the objective effect (the thrust or movement produced in the material), that eventually it may be recalled 'automatically' (i.e. without the intervention of the above-described processes) when it is desired to bring about this effect.

(d) *Cognizing 'anticipatory' characters.* The mental processes here are similar to those involved in cognizing the spatial arrangement of the fingers. The change introduced constitutes a new character in this spatial arrangement, which is now educed not merely in relation to the immediately ensuing movement but also in regard to the anticipated difficulty. The difficulty itself is usually directly apprehended in the course of experience as certain characters of the finger movements which must be avoided in future.

---

[1] Technically, with the spatial characters of the movement imparted to the material.
[2] The efforts made by the right hand and by the left, when, as in this case, they are interdependent and simultaneous, are regarded as one complex movement.

PART V

GENERAL SUMMARY

CHAPTER XVI

THE MAJOR CONCLUSIONS AND THEIR SIGNIFICANCE

A. THE ORGANIZATION OF MANUAL SKILL

1. THE PROBLEM OF MENTAL ORGANIZATION.

We have now traversed the whole of the ground which we set out to cover in this inquiry. In this final chapter we shall review our main conclusions and examine briefly their significance for current psychological theory and practice.

We began with a general study of engineering work, for the writer had already carried out an extensive inquiry into certain aspects of this work associated with mechanical aptitude. The variety and importance of manual activities in many branches of human endeavour, and a lack of precise psychological knowledge respecting many of these activities, suggested that a closer study of this field might yield fruitful results. A review of the relevant literature, coupled with first-hand observation of many kinds of manual work, led to a concentration of our inquiry on that form of manual activity called popularly, but with little regard for scientific accuracy, 'assembling work'; for it was seen not only that the mental and manual operations commonly included under the term 'assembling' occupied a place in industry sufficiently important to warrant careful study on their own account, but that they also offered many problems of wider psychological interest and of fundamental importance.

Not least among these problems is that which forms the main topic of the second part of this book, namely, the problem of mental organization. The implications of this problem, and its practical importance in the sphere of mental measurement, were discussed in our first chapter. There we saw that valid inferences respecting human 'abilities' demanded an objective analysis of mind in terms of unitary 'factors' and their functional relations. In Chapter II we saw, further, that the activities which we proposed to analyse were broadly divisible into two classes—namely, those requiring only manual skill, which we called 'routine assembling' (including 'stripping'), and those requiring, in addition, the solution of the problem as to how the parts to be assembled go together. These, following previous usage, we called 'mechanical assembling' operations. Later on, in order to extend our knowledge of important factors disclosed in the analysis of the routine assembling operations, a third group of activities was examined. These were simpler manual operations than those involved in routine assembling, of a kind frequently used as tests of manual dexterity.

With these broad distinctions and the results of previous researches in mind, the specific questions in this part of our inquiry were formulated as follows:

(1) How far does the general factor (general intelligence, or more precisely 'g'), which has been found[1] to enter into all kinds of mental (cognitive) activities, enter, as a determinant of success, into these assembling activities?

(2) How far does the mechanical factor (more precisely 'm'), which has been found[2] to enter into the mental activities involved in solving mechanical problems, extend its influence to assembling operations?

(3) What other factors determine success in assembling operations?

(4) How, with respect to 'factors', are the simpler manual operations related to the more complex assembling operations?

2. The problem of mental measurement.

In order to answer these questions, it was necessary to secure suitable measures of ability in the activities to be investigated. Hence, our inquiry opened with a study of the reliability of the measurements upon which our conclusions must ultimately rest. This we have dealt with in detail in Chapter IV. It included a study of the conditions under which reliable measures may be best secured, and of the influences affecting test scores. The results arrived at indicated a degree of

---

[1] By C. Spearman, in *The Abilities of Man* (London: Macmillan, 1927).

[2] By the present writer, see *Mechanical Aptitude* (London: Methuen, 1928).

accuracy in our tests sufficient to warrant their subsequent use as measures of ability, and that many of our findings respecting the influences affecting 'reliability' appear to have a wide and direct bearing on the practice of mental measurement in general. Especially interesting, in this connection, are (i) the observed increase in the reliability of a mental measurement which was brought about by increasing the number of samples of the individual's performance, (ii) the absence of any marked influence of practice on reliability so long as the sample of performance was taken at the same stage of practice for all individuals, (iii) the dependence of reliability on the number of repetitions constituting the measure, rather than on the length or complexity of the operation measured, and (iv) the general similarity between the reliability of our measures of ability in routine assembling operations and the accuracy with which they would predict ability after practice at the operation.

3. THE BROAD 'ABILITIES'.

Since 'ability' is a common term in psychology, and much may be gained from a study of an 'ability', pending knowledge of the more precisely determined 'factors' which underlie it, it would seem useful to summarize our findings with respect to the abilities examined in this inquiry. But, before doing so, we would remind the reader of the sense in which we use the term 'ability'. We have used this term in the popular sense, as when a person says he is able to do such and such a thing; and the evidence of the existence of his proclaimed ability is provided by his actually doing it, and is measured by the success he attains in the doing. In this sense every operation measured in our inquiry is an 'ability' and is measured by the success achieved in performing it, as indicated by the score made in the test.

The popular mind, finding it too hampering to pay strict regard to the almost infinite number of abilities of which man may be capable, tends to group them into broad classes, according to their more or less superficial resemblances. Thus, in common parlance, we speak of 'engineering ability', meaning the ability to perform the various activities required of an engineer. More frequently, it is the accomplished product (such as a poem) that is first noticed, and this gives rise to the notion of an existent correlative 'ability' (such as 'poetic ability'), without prior direct reference to any class of activities.

The activities we have investigated fall into three broad groups according to the sort of ability which, in the above popular sense, they seemed to require. Thus the tests of general intelligence and the examination in general school subjects form an 'intelligence' group; the mechanical aptitude tests and the mechanical assembling tests form a 'mechanical' group; and the routine tests form a 'manual' group. If now, following popular usage, we postulate three corresponding 'abilities', viz. 'general intelligence', 'mechanical ability' and 'manual ability', it would be fallacious to suppose that these exist as independent mental qualities. That such is not the case is clear from our studies of the inter-correlations of these groups of activities, described in Chapter v. Further observation also suggests the probability of some overlapping, for the mechanical group of tests is divisible into (*a*) a group in which manual work is absent (the mechanical aptitude tests), and (*b*) a group which involves manual work as well as mechanical problems (the mechanical assembling tests); and the manual group is divisible into (*a*) activities sufficiently complex as to render them not entirely unlike the mechanical assembling tests, namely, the routine assembling operations, (*b*) the stripping operations, which, while using the same material, were less likely to involve a 'mechanical' ability, and (*c*) the simple manual operations where anything akin to 'mechanical' operations seemed entirely foreign.

It was the purpose of our inter-correlational studies in Chapter v to determine how far this grouping of 'abilities', or 'functions', as we preferred to call them, was justified in practice. Our results have shown that neither the individual members of the group, nor any group as a whole, can be regarded as an independent 'ability' such as is implied in popular usage of this term. On the contrary, the various activities are inter-related; but the relationships are closer in some cases than in others, and some activities enter into wider and more complicated relationships than do others. Thus the activities grouped together above as 'intelligent', 'mechanical', or 'manual' are more closely related to other members of the same group than to members of the other groups.

In the 'mechanical' group, the mechanical aptitude tests are more closely related to one another than to the mechanical assembling tests. The latter are, if anything, more closely related to the aptitude type of test than to one another. In the 'manual' group, the corresponding relationship tends to become closer as the operations become more complex, and as the measures of ability become more exhaustive.

Thus, this part of our inquiry showed that the above grouping of activities into three broad 'abilities' was, at best, only approximate, and called for closer analysis of the data to determine whether the observed relations were statistically significant and, if so, how they could be best explained.

4. THE UNDERLYING 'FACTORS'.

The necessary statistical instruments for this analysis were provided by Spearman's method of tetrad differences and Yule's method of partial correlation, as described in Chapters VI–VIII. It will be remembered that a 'factor' was distinguished by definition from an 'ability', as an underlying influence, or cause, which partly determines ability but which, unlike an 'ability', functions as a unitary whole and in independence of other factors. The factors which we sought in this part of our inquiry were thus the functional elements into which the activities measured by our tests could be most usefully analyzed for purposes of mental measurement.

In the course of this analysis, the following factors were disclosed as best accounting for the observed inter-relations of the various activities: (i) a general factor which functions throughout the whole of the activities, with the possible exception of the simplest manual operations, (ii) a 'mechanical' factor of more restricted range, which functions only in those activities which involve a mechanical problem (e.g. the mechanical aptitude and the mechanical assembling tests), (iii) a 'routine manual' factor, restricted to the routine assembling and stripping operations and the simple manual tests, and (iv) two small additional factors each restricted to a pair of the simple manual tests involving closely similar movements.

In addition to these general and group-factors, there appears to be a further determinant of ability, namely a factor peculiar to each operation, i.e. one which enters into no other operation. This specific factor plays a relatively larger part in some of the simpler manual activities involved in the routine stripping operations and in the simple manual tests.

5. SATURATION.

Having located the factors, our final step was to determine their magnitude. 'Saturation' coefficients were, accordingly, calculated, showing the correlation between each factor and the activities into which it entered. These indicate that the general factor enters more into the mechanical aptitude tests than into either the mechanical assembling tests or the routine assembling tests, and least of all into the stripping tests.

As compared with the specific factors, the general factor enters into the 'mechanical' group of tests to a less extent than does the mechanical factor, and similarly, in the routine assembling groups, the general factor plays a smaller part than the specific 'routine manual' factor.

So much for their *relative influence*. As regards *degree*, the mechanical group of tests is more highly saturated with its 'mechanical' factor than is the routine manual group with its 'routine manual' factor; and, within the group, the 'aptitude' tests are more highly saturated with the mechanical factor than are the mechanical assembling tests. The more complex routine assembling tests likewise excel over the simple stripping tests with respect to the 'routine manual' factor. It follows that the 'aptitude' and the 'routine assembly' types of test are likely to yield the better measures of their respective group-factors.

6. SIGNIFICANCE OF THE ANALYSIS.

(*a*) *For psychological theory.* Theories regarding the way mind functions are of three kinds. According to one, success at all forms of human endeavour is wholly determined by one and the same trait, such as 'intelligence' or 'brains'. A second theory views the mind as organized into 'faculties', each of which functions independently of the others, and wholly determines success at the particular form of endeavour that calls it into play. A third theory postulates a large number of psychological elements which function in complete independence of one another.

Our results support none of these views in an extreme form, but find an element of truth in all three. The general factor is akin to the single trait of the first of these theories, but it does not operate alone, for with it are the group-factors, themselves somewhat akin to the faculties in their broad scope, but entirely different in operating simultaneously with the general factor; while each specific factor peculiar to a particular activity is comparable to one of the independent elements of the third theory. The present results support and extend the conclusions reached in a previous research in a cognate field.[1]

(*b*) *For mental measurement.* The location and measurement of the

---

[1] See *Mechanical Aptitude, loc. cit.*

factors in our data are of more than theoretical interest. The 'factors', as we have seen, provide a more fundamental and satisfactory basis for the analysis and classification of vocational aptitudes than do 'abilities'. It is evident that tests intended to measure a *special* aptitude can only succeed in proportion as the influences determining the score at the test are (i) the same as those which determine the aptitude, and (ii) enter into both test and aptitude in a 'special' way, i.e. as specific or group-factors. This is precisely the kind of knowledge provided by the 'factor' analysis.

Of the two broad group-factors disclosed in our data, one had already been discovered by the writer in his mechanical aptitude tests. Its intrusion into mechanical assembling operations as the same 'mechanical' factor had not been established before. Its greater potency in the aptitude tests and in the more difficult mechanical assembling tests provides an important indication for its measurement. The small part played by the 'routine manual' factor in mechanical assembling hardly justifies the practice of using such tests to measure both the 'mechanical' and the 'manual' factors simultaneously. In these, the manual activity functions specifically and so fails to provide a more general measure.

The 'manual' factor is a new discovery so far as the writer is aware. Its extension through the routine assembling and stripping tests to the simple tests suggests that it is of wide range. At the same time, the specific factor is the major determining influence in the simpler tests.

(c) *For vocational and educational guidance.* We have discussed at some length elsewhere[1] the importance of a knowledge of the factors underlying engineering occupations, more especially in relation to the 'mechanical' factor. There we have suggested a classification of these occupations, and of technical school subjects, according to their 'saturation' with the 'mechanical' factor. Similar remarks would seem to apply with respect to the 'routine manual' factor. The increase of 'saturation' with complexity, the tendency for the group-factor to disappear in the simpler manual operations and for new factors of small range to appear in closely similar activities, carry with them important suggestions for the classification and measurement of the many manual operations which enter so largely into the work of the factory and into the practical side of technical skill. In the sphere of assembling work, the results are of immediate application in indicating the nature

---

[1] In *Mechanical Aptitude*, see p. 5.

and scope of the more important factors and the kind of tests that best measure them. The closer association of the 'routine manual' factor with the more complex manual operations would seem to have an important bearing on manual training, indicating that breadth of training is to be looked for in complexity and variety rather than in simple repetition.

B. THE DEVELOPMENT OF MANUAL SKILL

1. THE MAIN PROBLEMS.

The second part of our inquiry was concerned with the development of skill in various manual operations, first under conditions of practice and then under conditions of formal training. The main problems fall into two broad classes: (i) how are the changes in ability brought about by practice related to one another? and (ii) under what conditions does the development of skill in one manual operation transfer to other operations?

The changes in ability for which data were secured included the total and percentage improvement made by each individual, and his variation in ability from day to day. These dynamic functions were compared with one another, with various measures of ability and with general intelligence. The curves of practice of many individuals and for many operations were also secured and examined.

The conditions under which the transference of manual skill was examined were: (i) those of 'practice', in which the subject repeated the operation at maximum speed; and (ii) those of 'training', in which the subject received instruction in the general principles underlying the development of manual skill and carried out formal exercises based on these principles.

2. THE CHANGES IN ABILITY WITH PRACTICE.

The practice curves were examined in considerable detail in Chapter x, and their general features have been summarized there. Among the more interesting of these is the tendency of the practice curve to divide into (*a*) a relatively short initial phase of steep slope which appears more closely associated with the cognitive side of the manual operation, followed by (*b*) a longer phase of more gradual descent, which seems more closely associated with the motor side. The tendency for individuals to maintain the same relative positions as practice continued, notwithstanding that individual differences diminish in magnitude, is of obvious import where manual tests are to be employed to predict individual improvability. The same may be said of the tendency for marked daily variability to be associated with weak ability.

The tendency for weaker individuals to make greater progress than those who start at a higher level, and the tendency for the practice curves to flatten into straight lines, appear features which distinguish 'manual' learning from the more purely 'mental' forms.

Seeing that 'intelligence', as shown by school attainment, is too often the only criterion adopted for the selection of manual workers, its relation to ability and to improvability in the manual activities practised by our subjects is of practical interest. Our results show that, although 'general intelligence' is a better criterion than none at all, it is a poor one as compared with that afforded by the scores made at the more complex manual operations.

3. THE TRANSFERENCE OF MANUAL SKILL.

One of the most important questions associated with problems of mental organization and development is that relating to the manner in which the acquisition of skill in one kind of activity affects ability at other kinds. In this inquiry, two ways of developing skill were carefully distinguished and investigated. In one series of experiments, the skill was developed by repetition of the operation at maximum speed. In the second series, a specially devised scheme of training, which aimed at giving the subject insight into the best way to use his fingers, took the place of this more or less mechanical repetition. The very important differences attendant upon these two methods of developing skill, which the data in Chapters xi and xiii have brought out so clearly, have an obvious bearing on all forms of training, and especially on manual training.

That the skill developed by the practice afforded in the first series of experiments virtually fails to transfer to operations subsequently undertaken, is the more striking in view of the range and complexity of the manual activities investigated. These results conform with, and extend to, more complex activities, the conclusions arrived at by previous workers with respect to simpler manual operations.

In sharp contrast with the narrow effects of mere practice, were the broad and far-reaching effects of the training, given in the second series of experiments. For these were manifested not only in the superior ability shown by the trainees in every operation for which they were subsequently measured, but also in their superior rate of progress, as practice continued. This latter, dynamic, aspect of the effects of training would seem to merit closer study than it has hitherto received.

4. THE ACQUISITION OF SKILL.

The virtual failure of practice effects to transfer to other operations implies that skill so acquired does not represent an increase in the 'routine manual' factor, for this was involved in both the practised and the unpractised operations. It suggests that the acquisition of skill depends on (i) innate ability, determined largely by the routine factor and the general factor, and (ii) the specific experience, provided in the practice, upon which this works. Whereas the former is brought to all operations and is more akin to 'power', the latter differs from one operation to another and provides the 'material' to which the 'power' is applied. The clearer knowledge of the specific experience, which comes through practice, brings with it a finer and more rapid discrimination of the particular sensori-motor items involved in the operation, and a more or less conscious identification, and subsequent recognition, of those essential to success. As a result, the necessary movements become more finely adjusted and more rapidly made.

It is thus made clear why skill, acquired under 'practice' conditions, fails to transfer. Mere knowledge of the sensori-motor experiences associated with one manual operation conveys little about those relevant to another, in much the same way as knowledge of geographical facts conveys little knowledge about history. In the case of 'training', conditions were different, because this aimed at making clear not merely, or primarily, the items of experience, not merely their attributes ('characters'), as they occurred in the actual presentation, but rather the *general character* of their (relevant) attributes and of the appropriate response. The analogous case in teaching would be *how to study* geography. In 'practice', the relevant items came tardily and not always clearly to consciousness, whereas in 'training' their entry into the cognitive field was speeded up and accompanied by knowledge which enabled the trainee to distinguish the relevant from the irrelevant.

The 'practice' of our first series of experiments tends to shade off into the 'training' of our second series, according to the psychological knowledge with which the 'practiser' starts and his psychological ability to apply it to the manual activity. Usually, however, the learning acquired by 'practice' seldom goes beyond knowing *how* to use the fingers with more or less skill in a specific way, and the additional *why* imparted in 'training' is discovered only by psychological analysis.

C. THE MENTAL PROCESSES IN MANUAL SKILL

The training referred to above was based upon a subjective analysis of the manual operations. A detailed account of the mental activity involved in these is given in Part IV, where the processes are described and illustrated. Reference to the detailed table of contents will indicate the general course of the analysis and the main topics dealt with in this part of our investigation.

In our first chapter we referred to the serious gap in our knowledge of the psychological processes underlying manual activity. There we had reason to complain that the accounts contained in current literature seldom went beyond the descriptive level; and, even then, did not describe psychological processes. We saw that progress in the understanding and in the use of manual tests called for a closer analysis of the mental operations involved, and one in which the unitary mental processes essential to these operations were made clear. This, by the aid of Spearman's principles of cognition, we have endeavoured to supply.

The analysis divides into two parts. The first, described in Chapter XIV, elucidates the cognitive processes involved in the solution of the mechanical problem which accompanies certain forms of manual activity.[1] It attempts to disclose those processes which seem especially associated with the mechanical factor. It thereby extends to manual operations the analysis of mechanical aptitude which the writer has described in a previous book.[2] In the former analysis, the mechanical problems were of a quite different form, and were uncomplicated by manual activity. They related to the understanding and invention of mechanisms. The present extension of the analysis to include manipu-

---

[1] The mechanical assembling operations.
[2] *Op. cit.* p. 5.

lative operations throws light on another large class of engineering occupations.

Our analysis also includes an examination of the processes underlying the cognition of shape, and a discussion of these in relation to the child mind, and to drawing and design. The results are, therefore, of vocational interest, wherever the worker is called upon to deal with spatial material. In their bearing on the 'Gestalt' problem, it is hoped that they may also prove of general psychological interest.

The second part of the analysis deals with those manual activities which involve no special mechanical problem and which we have termed 'routine assembling' operations. It attempts to unravel the cognitive processes associated with the manual factor which our objective measurements disclosed. It includes an account of the kind of knowledge which is acquired by practice at manual operations, and an analysis, into elementary processes, of the mental activity essential to its acquisition. It is suggested that ability to carry out the cognitive processes there described is associated with the 'routine manual' factor which determines success at this kind of work, while the items of experience with which these processes deal (Spearman's 'fundaments') are provided in the course of practice.

The 'mechanical' factor and the 'routine' factor appear to enter into many occupations. The analytical results should, therefore, find a wide application in the field of vocational psychology. It is hoped that the methods of analysis here adopted may be usefully applied to other forms of manual work. The present attempt is the first of its kind, so far as the writer is aware. For these reasons the results may perhaps claim an interest and importance extending beyond the particular manual operations to which they relate.

INDEX

For EU product safety concerns, contact us at Calle de José Abascal, 56–1°,
28003 Madrid, Spain or eugpsr@cambridge.org.